Overcoming Barriers to Progress in Psychotherapy

This accessible guide comprehensively addresses why psychotherapy of diverse forms often falters and provides effective strategies to succeed.

Psychotherapy on occasion does not progress as both the client and therapist would like it to, and affecting deep-lasting change can be difficult and elusive. By addressing the spectrum of reasons for this occurrence inclusive of client, therapist, and interactive influences, barriers to psychotherapy progress can be managed, optimizing outcomes for the wellbeing of clients and success of psychotherapists. Given that the client, therapist, and interaction between both parties is integral to psychotherapy, coverage is provided in three sections: client influences, therapist influences, and interactive influences. Within each chapter, relevant literature is reviewed, key sources of the barrier to psychotherapy presented, and strategies for addressing the problem provided, with several case examples and vignettes.

This book is essential for psychotherapists of all backgrounds, including students of psychotherapy.

Brad Bowins is a psychotherapist, psychiatrist, researcher, and founder of the Centre for Theoretical Research in Psychiatry and Clinical Psychology.

Overcoming Barriers to Progress in Psychotherapy

A Clinician's Guide

Brad Bowins

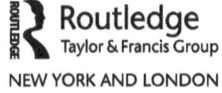
Routledge
Taylor & Francis Group

NEW YORK AND LONDON

Designed cover image: © Getty Image

First published 2023
by Routledge
605 Third Avenue, New York, NY 10158

and by Routledge
4 Park Square, Milton Park, Abingdon, Oxon, OX14 4RN

Routledge is an imprint of the Taylor & Francis Group, an informa business

© 2023 Brad Bowins

ISBN: 978-1-032-51254-9 (hbk)
ISBN: 978-1-032-44453-6 (pbk)
ISBN: 978-1-003-40137-7 (ebk)

DOI: 10.4324/b23346

Typeset in Garamond
by KnowledgeWorks Global Ltd.

This book is dedicated to all those who have benefited from or provided psychotherapy.

Contents

Preface

Psychotherapy is the most common type of intervention for mental illness when the full spectrum of problems is considered. Many clients have benefited enormously, suffering transformed into healthy functioning. Unfortunately, progress is often limited with approximately one-third dropout rates an indicator. For the two-thirds of clients who persist with psychotherapy, less-than-ideal outcomes are fairly common, generating frustration and disappointment for both the consumer and therapist. The combination of solid potential and real limitations necessitates an exploration of factors impeding the progress of psychotherapy, and application of robust strategies to reduce dropout rates and enhance outcomes.

Considering both the numerous forms of psychotherapy practiced and mental health conditions treated, comprehensive coverage of impediments to psychotherapy progress is challenging. Frequently, the coverage is restricted to hindrances particular to a form of psychotherapy, such as the completion of homework assignments in cognitive therapy. While important within the given form of therapy, such coverage restricts our overall understanding of the topic and efforts to improve the success of psychotherapy. *Overcoming Barriers to Progress in Psychotherapy: A Clinician's Guide* comprehensively addresses why psychotherapy of diverse forms often falters and provides effective across therapy strategies to improve outcomes. Given that the client, therapist, and interaction between both parties is integral to psychotherapy, coverage is provided in three sections:

Client Influences
* Motivation
* Expectations
* Personality Disorders
* Reinforcement Parameters
* Complexity
* Resistance and Noncompliance
* Impaired States and Processes for Mental Health
* Transference

Therapist Influences
- Countertransference
- Emotional Factors
- Personality Factors
- Skill Factors

Interactive Influences
- Therapeutic Alliance
- Interactions Between Client and Therapist Influences

Within each chapter the relevant literature is reviewed, key sources of the given psychotherapy impediment presented, and strategies for addressing the problem provided, with case examples where illustrative. Beyond including client, therapist, and interactive factors impeding the progress of psychotherapy, the coverage is novel in the following ways:

First, most books pertaining to psychotherapy hindrances work from a set theoretical perspective, an occurrence that can limit how applicable the content is to the spectrum of psychotherapy scenarios. In the current book, barriers to psychotherapy progress are examined from diverse and comprehensive perspectives, ensuring that the material spans the range of therapies and mental health conditions. This treatment of barriers to psychotherapy progress does not negate the value of approaches focused on a specific form of psychotherapy, instead adding to such strategies.

Second, efforts to understand what blocks progress in psychotherapy often emphasize resistance and noncompliance, both characterized by a negative client-based focus. On a more positive note, it does seem that the majority of prospective clients have the potential to substantially improve with psychotherapy, or why even consider it and attend for an assessment? Hence, the more hopeful perspective is taken that most clients do have the potential to advance with psychotherapy, while acknowledging and addressing profound impediments to psychotherapy progress.

Third, in line with the positive and hopeful focus, there is a coverage of states and processes for mental health. Activity, psychological defense mechanisms, social connectedness, psychological regulation, human specific cognition (executive functions, social cognition, and motivation), self-acceptance, and adaptability characterize mental health and optimize positive affect. Impairments to these states and processes produce mental illness and impede psychotherapy progress. Strategies to advance these states and processes to achieve more optimal psychotherapy outcomes are indicated.

Fourth, where appropriate techniques are provided which clients can apply to overcome barriers to psychotherapy progress. This component is important because although many treatments of the topic focus on client factors, strategies are only generated for the therapist! Given that both the client and therapist play a role in psychotherapy outcomes, active participation of the client is important for their empowerment and progress. These client techniques can either be suggested by the therapist or sought directly by the client.

Based on my experience as a psychotherapist and research studies, it is clear that psychotherapy does not always progress as both the client and therapist would like it to. Effecting change can be difficult and elusive. However, by addressing the spectrum of reasons for this occurrence inclusive of client, therapist, and interactive influences, diverse impediments to psychotherapy progress can be managed, thereby reducing dropout rates and optimizing outcomes for the well-being of clients and success of psychotherapists. Given the across therapy orientation, psychotherapists and students of diverse theoretical backgrounds can benefit. Although the content is focused on individual psychotherapy, the client, therapist, and interactive barriers to psychotherapy progress also apply to couple, family, and group therapy.

Acknowledgment

The insightful feedback from Dr. Irwin Kleinman derived from his review of the book is greatly appreciated.

About the Author

Brad Bowins is a psychotherapist, psychiatrist, researcher, and founder of the Centre for Theoretical Research in Psychiatry and Clinical Psychology. His research and writings challenge the status quo, fostering paradigm shifts so crucial to the progression of science and knowledge. Several theoretical perspectives, presented in peer-reviewed papers and books, have advanced the way that key aspects of mental illness and psychotherapy are understood. Extensive frontline work by Dr. Bowins ensures that the theories align with clinical realities. Consistent with the notion that there is nothing so practical as a good theory, novel and effective psychotherapy interventions for mental illness follow from the theoretical advances. Based on the combination of extensive experience providing psychotherapy and conducting relevant research, the practical and conceptual aspects of barriers to psychotherapy progress represent an ideal fit, with the resulting therapeutic strategies applicable by psychotherapists.

Section I

Client Influences

Chapter 1

MOTIVATION

Without motivation, or very little motivation, progress in any endeavor is impeded. If I am not motivated to learn the piano, how can I possibly progress? Of course, there is internal (intrinsic) and external (extrinsic) motivation that both play a role. Maybe, I have to learn the piano to graduate from a music class, so there is some motivation despite my lack of intrinsic motivation. Regarding psychotherapy, clients typically have some motivation, at least if extrinsic motivation is taken into account, or why even present for an assessment and then enter into psychotherapy? However, the degree of motivation is a major concern, and certainly relative to the costs. We will look at client motivation considering the benefit/cost ratio, intrinsic and extrinsic motivation, and motivation to change. In addition to client motivation, therapist motivation might be an issue, but it is predominately client based, given that a therapist is significantly motivated to provide psychotherapy, or why select this profession at all and remain in it? At the very least there will be a financial motivation, unless the therapist is fortunate enough to be independently wealthy. Therapists also want to help people and believe in the power of psychotherapy, providing a more humanistic source of motivation. Therapists who lack these forms of motivation typically exit from their practice. Relevant to motivation for working with a given client is countertransference that will be covered in the Countertransference chapter. An interesting aspect of motivation relates to the interaction between the client and therapist, in that when a therapist perceives motivation in a client their own motivation is enhanced, setting up a positive interaction from the start. Coverage of motivation is provided first because it plays a major role in the success or failure of psychotherapy right from the start, and even prior to engaging.

BENEFIT/COST RATIO

I am framing it as benefit/cost, instead of the more typical cost/benefit to emphasize the positive value, and not a fraction, when benefits exceed costs—for instance, 9/3 as opposed to 3/9. There are numerous potential benefits and also costs associated with psychotherapy. The assumption is that when benefits

DOI: 10.4324/b23346-2

substantially exceed costs for a given endeavor motivation is robust. I will now list some of potential benefits and costs of psychotherapy, based on discussions with clients and what I have observed. The lists for potential benefits and costs are much more extensive than what is provided here, given that many influences, including emotional, personal, relationship, cultural, and highly individualistic, can enter the picture.

Benefits
- Feeling better.
- Understanding myself.
- Less focused on negative things.
- More success in relationships.
- Improved capacity to cope.
- Career success or at least overcoming stagnation.
- Self-respect.
- Less guilt.
- Capacity to understand others.
- Dealing with trauma.
- Not so isolated.
- Less anger.

Costs
- Financial aspect, relevant in most parts of the world.
- Time commitment.
- Fear of change.
- Painful self-discovery.
- Having to face difficult issues.
- Approaching feared situations.
- Accepting flaws.
- Realizing that I have wasted time or my life.
- Becoming more aware of regrets.

Addressing both potential benefits and costs to psychotherapy will assist in identifying the level of client motivation. McEvoy and Nathan (2007) examining 173 psychotherapy clients with anxiety and affective disorders, found that those who acknowledged both sides of the equation achieved better outcomes than those only or mostly focused on benefits. This result is interesting given the increased ambivalence compared to only or mostly seeing beneficial aspects of psychotherapy. It seems feasible that appreciating both benefits and costs contributes to a solid and sustainable level of motivation. If a person only or mostly acknowledges benefits, the costs will start to become apparent as therapy proceeds, reducing motivation. I have encountered this with clients who enter only focused on what psychotherapy will help them with. As costs both practical such as missed session payments, and psychological as with facing difficult issues are incurred motivation declines, and it usually plays out much better if motivation based on a solid benefit/cost ratio remains stable or increases during therapy.

Assuming that motivation based on the benefit/cost ratio is important what can be done about it?

Therapist Role

Certain questions will get the client thinking about their motivation for psychotherapy. I find that a helpful general question is "What are you hoping to get from psychotherapy?" Open ended questions are best as they encourage thought and elicit more information. If a client presents solid goals like those mentioned above under the heading Benefits, then it is a safe assumption that there is sufficient motivation. If the person draws a blank or really struggles with it, examples of possible goals can help, but a therapist has to be careful of creating goals that are not there. If the person is still not responding well, then address perceived costs such as: "What costs do you see as being involved?" If the client readily presents several, then it is likely that perceived costs exceed perceived benefits, and motivation is limited. An advantage of this approach is addressing concerns head-on. For example, "I'm afraid of becoming a different person." A helpful response consists of, "A person always retains their core personality, while learning to be more successful with it." Such responses often produce a noticeable sense of relief, and the prospective client will then open up about other fears pertaining to psychotherapy. In some instances, asking about perceived costs elicits information that can be a deal breaker for psychotherapy. For example, "I believe more in homeopathic medicine, but my family doctor suggested this, and I did not want to upset her." Trying to "sell" psychotherapy will not help, and responding in a more benign fashion is usually best. For example, "Different approaches can be helpful and the choice is yours, but would you like me to give you an overview of psychotherapy so you know what it offers?" In other words, do not challenge a person on their views. I have seen prospective clients warm up, or call back a few weeks later indicating that they have reconsidered psychotherapy and wish to try it.

An important issue is the timing of questions pertaining to benefits and costs. I suggest at the end of the assessment, or at least the first assessment session for therapists who take more than one session to complete it. The reason being that the assessment process itself will often elicit information relevant to motivation, such as fear of becoming a different person, that can be addressed on the spot. Assessments also get the client thinking about their issues enabling them to see potential benefits, and maybe even costs. An example of the latter is, "I am so busy and am not sure that I have the time for this." Responding on the spot such as, "Psychotherapy can help people become more efficient with their time, and feel more empowered," addresses their concern.

In some instances, concerns about psychotherapy arise pre-assessment, such as during the initial telephone contact, and then have to be managed at this point.

Client ratings of benefits and costs is a more advanced way of addressing the benefit/cost ratio. From experience, I have found that 1–10 (or 1–5, 1–7) ratings can be helpful in assessing various parameters, such as, "On a 1–10 scale with 1 the lowest and 10 the highest, how do you rate your mood on average over the last month?" This rating process readily applies to benefits and costs. Have the client rate both perceived benefits and costs to psychotherapy on separate scales. If the person struggles to see what might apply under each, examples can be given from the lists provided above. This rating can be done on the spot, an advantage being that it elicits true feelings. Another approach is to have the client complete it after the assessment and bring it in to discuss next session. An advantage of this second option is that the client has time to list perceived benefits and costs to make a more informed rating, and discuss these pluses and minuses the next session. Conceivably both options can be applied for an immediate emotional response and a more thought out consideration.

When the benefit/cost ratio is in the range of 6–10/1–5, then solid motivation exists. If the opposite range applies, as with 1–5/6–10, then the therapist might suggest to the client that their motivation is not optimal, and psychotherapy needs to be reconsidered. I take the approach, "Effort and time is involved to make this work, and your motivation does not seem optimal at the present time. Perhaps you want to take some time to think about it, and call me when ready." Besides empowering the client with the decision, an additional advantage is that in some instances the prospective client might have concerns about the therapist that cannot be altered, and has the option of looking for another therapist. For example, the client might be young and the therapist older, and the person wants a therapist who will be there for years. While it is true that addressing this concern can yield positive outcomes, such as the therapist explaining that they have no plans of retiring and wish to work for many more years, the reality is often that the client feels uncomfortable discussing something that cannot be altered, and it is best to let the person think about it. I have even had a couple of very young clients return saying that they were concerned about this, but feel that the connection is more important than age and so decided to proceed.

Therapists can encourage prospective clients to discuss perceived benefits and costs. If more costs than benefits are presented and the assessment reveals a clear bias to negative thinking, this can be addressed such as, "From our discussion, it seems that you take a cup half empty perspective on most things, and you might be doing the same for psychotherapy." This type of feedback often assists a client in recalibrating their ratings, but if the person reacts negatively then it is a sign that therapy most likely will not proceed well, given that from the client's perspective costs exceed benefits, and the person might be too embedded in negative reactions to alter the ratio. Negative transference (covered in the Transference chapter) might also be an issue, and when such negativity strongly emerges during the assessment phase, combined with a perception that costs of psychotherapy will exceed benefits, it is usually an indicator that therapy is unlikely to proceed well, or will be a very uphill battle.

Some therapists just assume that a prospective client has high motivation given that the person has presented for psychotherapy, and then simply proceed without assessing motivation and concerns. While it is often true that those who present for an assessment are motivated with a robust benefit/cost ratio, this is not always the case, and can lead to problems including limited participation, missed sessions early in treatment, and withdrawal from therapy. This type of occurrence produces frustration and even anger on the part of the therapist, contributing to reduced career motivation and even burnout. I believe that it is far better to address the client's motivation in terms of perceived benefits and costs right at the start, to prevent or reduce the likelihood of negative occurrences.

Client Role

Prospective psychotherapy clients best consider their motivation level, assessing both perceived benefits and costs as described above on separate rating scales. This approach helps assess motivation and also clarifies goals. For example, the client might realize that the quality of their romances and friendships is an ongoing problem, that psychotherapy can address. Improving romances and friendships then becomes a salient goal. Likewise, the person might appreciate that they always view things in a negative fashion, perhaps even psychotherapy, and altering negative perspectives becomes a goal for psychotherapy. Clients who tend to take a cup half empty perspective on most things, best appreciate that they might be doing this for psychotherapy, leading to too low ratings for benefits and too high for costs. Recalibrating the ratings accordingly will help, and also be a focus for therapy.

Clients are then encouraged to consider their motivation for psychotherapy, both in terms of potential benefits and costs. Therapists can assist in this client role, by encouraging prospective clients to engage in this evaluation, and respond flexibly to any concerns. A special circumstance arises when motivation pertains to the type of therapy provided by the psychotherapist. For example, the client has been abused and traumatized, and the therapist practices cognitive behavioral therapy mostly for depression and anxiety. A very legitimate client concern pertaining to motivation is, does the type of psychotherapy fit with my issue? In this specific example, I have had several cognitive behavioral therapists refer clients when their intervention was failing, despite going well beyond the manual. The fit between client issue and type of psychotherapy was not a solid one, resulting in failure to progress. Based on my experience, I have come to believe in eclectic psychotherapy as it allows for the flexible provision of what works for a given client at a particular point in time. In some instances, a client will hold back from revealing abuse and later present it. A time-limited cognitive approach rarely cuts it at this point, and there needs to be a longer term intensive focus on the impact of trauma.

INTRINSIC AND EXTRINSIC MOTIVATION

Intrinsic refers to from within and extrinsic external sources of motivation. For the most part, client motivation for psychotherapy is intrinsic based on my experience, and derives from the type of benefits listed above. Extrinsic motivation takes the form of a court order for psychotherapy, requirement for continuation of employment or schooling, or a significant person (spouse, relative, friend) fed up with certain behavior. As an example of a work-based scenario, a middle age man, Sam (not his real name), had an interaction with a younger female employee who reported him for verbal assault. Sam had a history of being sexually and physically abused by his adoptive father, and experienced anger. My work with Sam started a few years earlier, initiated by escalating anxiety. He presented as calm during the initial assessment, but in the first few sessions of therapy expressed anger in his tone and challenging responses. Addressing emotions is usually the best strategy in this scenario and I raised the point, "You seem to be very angry at me, and I cannot recall saying anything to offend you." His reaction was much more striking than even I thought it might be. He looked shocked and then uttered, "I'm not aware of being angry towards you." Therapy then proceeded with interpreting the transference (see the Transference chapter), and showing how he perceives authority figures as not being trustworthy and likely to violate him, producing anger. He progressed well with this understanding and consciously examined his reaction to others. His work required him to interact with various individuals and feedback improved leading to good performance evaluations. What happened with this one junior employee was not clear, as he maintained he never threatened her, and even when demonstrating anger toward me I did not feel that he would attack verbally or physically. Perhaps her own background made her overly sensitive, combined with some anger in his expression. Regardless of the reality, he was required to continue psychotherapy (or start it if not involved), and he worked on this specific incident learning more about anger and ways to regulate it. He accepted that he can appear angry and potentially threatening, enhanced by his tall stature.

Court-ordered psychotherapy is an occurrence that I have had limited experience with, but within that restricted scenario I have seen a range of responses covering the spectrum, from going through the motions required to satisfy the court order, to working very hard on the pertinent issues. An example of the latter is a client I will call Tim, who triggered an automobile accident while intoxicated and was required to seek addiction counseling. He was remorseful about the event and worked very hard on understanding his behavior, such as how when stressed and experiencing negative emotions he numbed himself through alcohol. This often just made things worse, leading to more negative emotions, more drinking, worsening circumstances and emotions, and so on and so forth. He entered into Alcoholics Anonymous, in addition to addiction counseling, and despite a few brief relapses has led a clean and sober lifestyle, learning to work with negative emotions and circumstances. A type of "order" I have had more experience with pertains to university students, as for approximately for 10 years I worked part-time at University of Toronto Psychiatric Service. Students who had very negative interactions with professors or other students were in some instances required to seek counseling. This experience mirrored my more limited court-ordered psychotherapy work: some clients worked with the requirement utilizing the external motivation to improve, and others more or less went through the motions, with a range of responses encountered.

A major reason why I mention a range of client responses to extrinsic sources of motivation, is a persistent social psychology theme of extrinsic motivation undermining intrinsic motivation (Deci et al., 1999). This perspective maintains that external sources of motivation will reduce motivation already present arising from internal sources. I have some familiarity with this topic, because way back in a pre-med psychology course, I ran a small experiment based on this concept that was popular at the time. My project adhered to the standard protocol for eliciting the effect and utilized undergraduate students as subjects, standard back then and now, and it was incredibly difficult to even elicit this effect at all. Given that the methodology was sound, I came to believe that the undermining intrinsic motivation with extrinsic motivation effect was largely false. Over more recent history, the topic of research bias has moved to the forefront, with many seemingly established psychology principles not reproducible. My purpose here, given that this is a book about psychotherapy, is not to go over the largely intractable literature pertaining to extrinsic motivation undermining intrinsic motivation, but to reveal that in practice the concept is very weak.

Based on my psychotherapy experience, I cannot recall a clear example of an extrinsic source of motivation for psychotherapy undermining intrinsic motivation. What I have seen is summated and interactive motivation. For example, when a client's partner or employer suggests counseling, and the person acknowledges an issue, motivation is enhanced because there is a personal reason to address the problem given recognition of the concern, and also external reward such as maintaining and even advancing with the job or relationship. In some instances, these sources of motivation interact, such as, by addressing the problem in therapy self-concept and self-esteem are enhanced, which in turn empowers the person to progress further with the external issue. I have not experienced a person no longer caring about self-improvement due to an external source of motivation for psychotherapy. This aligns with the core sources of intrinsic motivation suggested by self-determination theory, as articulated by Deci and Ryan (2012), consisting of competency, autonomy, and relatedness. Other than potentially autonomy, which might conceivably appear to be threatened by external motivation, these core needs forming the basis of intrinsic motivation are quite resilient to any undermining influence of external forces. Regarding autonomy, consistent with self-determination theory, the autonomy of clients must be respected and fostered (Deci & Ryan, 2012; Ryan et al., 2010). Mandated psychotherapy is more likely to work well when the therapist acknowledges the legitimacy of the client's negativism, possibly because it supports their autonomy, and also dissociates from the order so as not to be perceived as part of it (Storch & Lane, 1989).

As pertains to what the therapist and client can do to work with intrinsic and extrinsic sources of motivation.

Therapist Role

Encourage the client to identify benefits of psychotherapy both internal and external. Mentioning that both sources need be considered will help the client recognize a wider range of pluses to psychotherapy. This might be phrased to the effect of: "When you think of potential benefits to psychotherapy, consider both personal ones, and those related to your relationships, and work/school." As mentioned, there is no downside in terms of the external ones undermining internal ones, and even at face value, it is ludicrous that +3 internal motivation and +3 external motivation, will cancel resulting in 0 motivation. Theoretically and practically, +3 internal motivation and +3 external motivation will result in +6 additive motivation, or even +9 interactive motivation for psychotherapy. A therapist can provide examples if a client is struggling to make the distinction between internal and external sources of motivation. In some regards, confusion is understandable given that there can be combined internal and external aspects such as feeling better and empowered by improved relationships and/or work/school capacity.

Motivation for psychotherapy then best encompasses internal and external sources, with an understanding that they are additive or interact for a multiplying effect, and extrinsic sources of motivation for psychotherapy rarely if ever undermine intrinsic sources. Supporting this perspective, I have found that for clients required to have counseling, identifying personal benefits often helps the person forget about the "forced" aspect of attending and make the most of the experience! One example of this is applying a cognitive approach to suspicious and even psychotic level thoughts, a frequent source of "ordered" psychotherapy. If a client is told that working with thoughts such as these can make them feel better, they are usually open to the option. Cognitive therapy for psychotic thoughts is based on the principle of normalization (Kingdon & Turkington, 1994; Landa et al., 2006), meaning that these thoughts occupy the extreme end of a range of cognitive distortions, and bringing them back into the normal range is the goal of therapy. To achieve this normalization,

I have the client first attempt to provide evidence of their belief. For instance, if other students are perceived to be undermining credibility with the professor, where is the proof? Invariably there is no evidence, and it is helpful to remind a client that evidence is required for a conviction. The second step is to have the person generate alternative perspectives, acknowledging (not challenging) their position as one possibility. Perhaps the other students are insecure and trying to please the professor. Maybe, parents are pressuring them to perform better than others. The student or students who seem most at fault might do this to all students, and not just the client. The more alternative options generated, the more balanced the client's perspective becomes and it dilutes the suspicious one. The third step is to experiment or test perspectives. The client might take the role of an observer watching how the other students act during class, and discover that the person suspected of undermining the client's credibility is insecure and doing the same to everyone. Even though psychotic level thinking is often perceived by clinicians to absolutely require antipsychotic medication, this technique is very effective, and I have had clients thank me for not treating them as "crazy." As a word of caution, when the beliefs are fully in the psychotic range combining this cognitive therapy approach with antipsychotic medication works best. Regardless of the particular problem that gave rise to the requirement for psychotherapy, when the client perceives psychotherapy as an opportunity for self-improvement the external "forced" aspect recedes, along with any anger and resistance derived from it.

Client Role

When considering the benefits to psychotherapy, consider personal and external sources of motivation, appreciating that a given scenario such as a romance can have combined internal and external aspects. Also appreciate that internal and external sources of motivation are typically additive, but can interact producing an even greater impact, whereas the scenario of external sources of motivation undermining internal sources is for the most part ludicrous, at least as far as psychotherapy is concerned. Identifying both internal and external sources of motivation assists in accepting the costs of psychotherapy.

MOTIVATION TO CHANGE

For some people, clients and therapists alike, change is a scary word, and for others, it represents an opportunity for progress and rewards. Since the therapist is doing what he or she routinely does—psychotherapy—motivation to change is more of an issue for the client. Even though it might not be framed in this fashion, every therapist has seen a range of client motivation to change, for better or worse. Key influences underlying a client's motivation to change consist of personality factors, fear, and rigid patterns of behavior.

Personality

Normal personality dimensions have been distilled from years of research, with the so-called "Big 5" identified by Costa and McCrae (1992) being most reliable. They include introversion: extroversion, neurotic-emotionally stable, open-closed to experience, agreeable-antagonism, and conscientious-negligence. Of greatest relevance to motivation for change is open-closed to experience. People range from very closed to experiences to highly novelty seeking, and even though a person's propensity in this regard can vary depending on the type of activity, such as music preferences compared to adventure activities, those who are more open to experience tend to be quite novelty seeking generally. It naturally follows that a person who is open to experience will be more motivated for change, including when entering psychotherapy. Research indicates that openness to experience is predictive of long-term progress in psychotherapy (Samuel et al., 2018). The same research study also found that conscientiousness is positively linked to psychotherapy progress, at least in terms of early engagement (Samuel et al., 2018). A study of 250 clients revealed that openness to psychotherapy during the pretreatment interview predicted positive treatment outcomes (Schneider & Klauer, 2001).

A person who is closed to novel experiences will have much less motivation to change. A client example that comes to mind is Brian, a retired businessman who presented with depression. Part of the reason for his depression was the loss of activities he was familiar with during his career, and hesitancy throughout his life to adopt new activities that could be rewarding and uplifting. Noting that he demonstrated negative perspectives pertaining to several issues, including his future and what he might do with it, I suggested and went over a cognitive approach. He took to this approach like virtually no other client. In a few months, his depression resolved and he entered into new activities generated from the positive outlook, despite his personality based tendency to not experiment with novel pursuits, these activities further bolstering his mood, ensuring that the depression did not return.

In terms of what the therapist and client can do:

Therapist Role

During the assessment and subsequent sessions try to get a feel for how the client rates on the Big 5 personality dimensions, and in particular open-closed to experience. This evaluation can often be made from the activities a person reveals: when a client describes a very routine and monotonous life, it is a safe assumption that the person is closed to experience, whereas a person reporting experimentation with sexual activities and adventure travel is very open to experience. A question that can be applied consists of: "On a scale of 1 to 10, with 1 the lowest and 10 the highest, where do you rate your typical desire for unique experiences?" The word, typical, is important, because if the client is currently depressed motivation for novel experiences might be rated low if taken in the moment, whereas it is typically high. If a client appears to be quite closed to experience, it is helpful for the therapist to frame psychotherapy in familiar and safe terms, such as, "Therapy is really about talking," "You proceed at the pace that feels comfortable, and I will not pressure you." In the case of clients who are quite open to experience, indicating that therapy is an exploration and journey can enhance motivation to participate and change.

Client Role

Prior to and during therapy consider where you rate on openness to unique experiences. If the answer is low, then motivation for change might be limited. View the psychotherapy experience as familiar in that it really is about talking, a behavior everyone is used to. The pace of progress and change is also up to you the client and no one should feel rushed to change faster than what they are comfortable with. A related issue is that no one changes their core personality features, an occurrence some people, and particularly those closed to experience, are hesitant about. Therefore, appreciate that you will not become a different person (personality shifting), but instead work better with your core personality.

Fear

A nasty four-letter word, more potent than other negative four-letter words, when it comes to change. Fear arises when a person unconsciously or consciously perceives threat or danger (see the Expectations chapter). There is an obvious survival value and fear is present in all primates and mammals at least. Humans appear somewhat unique though in amplifying fear. One of my early theoretical propositions (Bowins, 2004) is that the evolution of human intelligence has amplified emotions—the Amplification Effect—by making the cognitive activating appraisals underlying emotions more intensive, extensive, and adding a temporal dimension. Pertaining to fear, we think of the various ramifications of a threat, such as a negative performance appraisal at work, intensifying the negative emotion. For example, "My colleagues will find out and disrespect me," "My boss will always be watching what I do." We also extend the threat, such as, "If I performed poorly at this job, then I will do badly at others." Then there is replaying such thoughts over days, weeks, months, and even years. Through intensification, extension, and replaying thoughts over time, the emotion is amplified. In regard to fear this emotion amplification fosters anxiety, and in regard to sadness, depression, based on cognitive activating appraisals detecting losses (Bowins, 2004).

If a person fears change and amplifies the perception, then positive change is blocked or greatly impeded. Some people are very prone to amplifying fear, resulting in substantial anxiety with avoidance a common response.

Whereas the therapist views psychotherapy as an opportunity for the client to improve and advance, the fear-prone client views it as a threat. Numerous things can be feared about therapy, such as changing who I am, having to do things I do not want to, facing past issues, with the list virtually endless. So, what can be done?

Therapist Role

The assessment if done thoroughly will reveal that the person has anxiety issues. From this it follows that the client might be fearful of psychotherapy generally or specific aspects. Addressing this concern head-on is usually best, such as by asking, "Is there anything about psychotherapy that concerns or worries you?" Dealing with fears raised does tend to diminish or eliminate them, enhancing motivation for change. Another way of looking at this occurrence is that once the barrier of fear is removed positive change motivation can be expressed. Then have the client face fears related to change in psychotherapy in a graded way from least to most intense.

A different approach to overcoming fear of change is increasing motivation, essentially replacing negative fear-based motivation with positive change motivation. Motivational interviewing comprises a set of person-centered techniques designed to enhance motivation for change, via the four key processes of engaging, focusing, evoking, and planning (Miller & Rollnick, 2012). Engaging involves the therapist getting to know and understand the client in an empathic fashion to develop trust. Focusing consists of identifying areas that are important to the client that represent a challenge. Discrepancies between their current situation and desired outcome are noted that can be applied to motivate change. Evoking identifies reasons why the person wants to change, encouraging the client to come up with their own strategies for change. Planning involves helping the client develop an action plan and commitment to change. As with Person-Centered Therapy, the client is to design the change process to empower the individual (Miller & Rollnick, 2012). By focusing on change and the value to the client, the negative motivation of fear is replaced with positive motivation for change.

Client Role

A client need consider, Am I fearful or worried about entering into psychotherapy? If the answer is yes, then try to identify and write down the concerns. Resist any fear about expressing these concerns and present them during the assessment, or at the start of actual therapy. Something I routinely tell anxiety-prone clients is that in 9/10 instances the reality is not as bad as imagined, and for the 1/10 cases where it is, facing it usually plays out better. Seeing numerous clients fear countless things, this 9/10 scenario might best be viewed as a rule. Regarding the change process, face fears pertaining to change in a

graded fashion from least to most intense, and engage with motivational interviewing if practiced by the therapist. If not practiced by the therapist, at least
attempt to apply the strategies of focusing, evoking, and planning described
under Therapist Role.

Rigid Patterns of Behavior

Flexible behavior adapted to circumstances promotes solid change motivation
and good mental health, whereas rigid behavior not suited to current circumstances results in dysfunction and mental illness. Back in the 1950s, Albert
Ellis noted this occurrence and designed rational-emotive therapy to assertively address rigid dysfunctional behaviors blocking progression toward good
mental health (Ellis, 1980, 1991). This aligns with my own research, and the
proposition that non-traumatic patterns of behavior often arise from patterns
of behavior modeled by caregivers and internalized (Bowins, 2010). Hence, if
parents demonstrate a pattern of avoiding stressors and challenges a child often
internalizes this pattern, at least if there is a fit with personality, and repeats it
as a default response. These rigid dysfunctional patterns of behavior can play
out endlessly generating ongoing problems, largely because they block positive
change. Of relevance to the present focus, they translate into a demotivation
for change. As an example, Hank presented with relationship problems both in
the work setting and in his personal life. Raised by distant and uncaring parents, where distrust and deception was the norm, he internalized this pattern.
It played out resulting in relationship and career setbacks, the latter usually
linked to relationship problems on the job. Instead of being open about being
"gay" he led others to believe he was "straight" but they sensed a deception. He
deceived me and others about not completing his university degree. If aware of
this I would have suggested, guided, and supported him in completing it, and
consequently some of the career issues would have been remedied. Despite his
intelligent and my efforts to assist him, he persisted in deceptions and eventually ended up unemployed and unable to live in Toronto. There was very little
positive change.

   What therapists and clients can do about rigid dysfunctional patterns of
behavior.

Therapist Role

Identify these patterns and assertively address them in therapy. Following the
lead of Albert Ellis, this is a challenge that has to be focused on and repeated
despite resistance from the client. In the case of Hank, I tried to get him to face
his distrust of people and related to this, deception. Perhaps if I realized the
intensity and relevance of the pattern earlier and/or he could have remained in
Toronto and in therapy, we might have turned the corner on it. If a client persists in self-destructive rigid patterns of behavior, a therapist can question the

client directly about motivation to change, and if the response is not positive suggest that therapy ends. Sometimes this will make the client realize how serious the issue is and really consider addressing it.

Client Role

Be open to input regarding an inflexible dysfunctional pattern of behavior, and not self-blame as these patterns arise from early life circumstances. Appreciate that to alter a dysfunctional pattern of behavior, a person must consciously overlearn the alternative, or in other words practice the more adaptive option whenever possible. In Hank's case this would have meant trusting unless there was a clear objective reason not to, preferably agreed upon by the therapist, and routinely be open about issues such as sexual orientation and education. Eventually, the new adaptive pattern will replace the old dysfunctional one. When rigid dysfunctional patterns of behavior are shifted to flexible adaptive patterns motivation to change improves, fostering progress in psychotherapy.

Motivation for change is a crucial component of overall motivation for psychotherapy, with personality in terms of open-closed to experience, fear of change, and rigid dysfunctional patterns of behavior, particularly relevant. Unfortunately, when change motivation is impaired by one or more of these three influences progression in psychotherapy is impeded. Fortunately, efforts by both the therapist and client can shift functioning on closed to experience, fear of change, and rigid dysfunctional patterns of behavior, producing a solid motivation for change in psychotherapy. A client example consists of Sally, a young woman who suffered from depression. She leaned to the side of being more closed to experience, tended to be fearful of change, and demonstrated the rigid behavioral pattern of clinging to partners. Due to setbacks at work she felt that she could not continue in her business career. With the support of therapy and my addressing the various impediments to change, she was able to imagine and progress with a less stressful career option, thereby demonstrating greater openness to unique experiences. She learned that most of her fears were unfounded and hence approached challenges instead of avoiding them, and she relinquished her tight hold on partners trusting more in herself and those who are trying to help. Consequently, she established a new successful career in adult education, and in the process progressed with managing her mood problems, and has advanced in terms of self-confidence and self-esteem.

SUMMARY NOTE

Motivation is core to any successful endeavor including psychotherapy participation. Although there are many aspects of motivation relevant to psychotherapy, the benefit/cost ratio, intrinsic and extrinsic motivation, and motivation for change stand out. Regarding motivation for change, personality factors (open-closed to experience), fear, and rigid patterns of behavior are particularly important. By addressing the key influences, therapists and clients can optimize client motivation for psychotherapy. The effort expended in this regard during the assessment phase or at the start of sessions, can save a great deal of frustration and wasted time and other resources arising from failure to progress.

REFERENCES

Bowins, B. E. (2004). Psychological defense mechanisms: A new perspective. *American Journal of Psychoanalysis*, *64*, 1–26.

Bowins, B. E. (2010). Repetitive maladaptive behavior: Beyond repetition compulsion. *American Journal of Psychoanalysis*, *70*, 282–298.

Costa, P. T., & McCrae, R. R. (1992). *Revised NEO personality (NEO-PI-R) and NEO five factor inventory (NEO-FFI) professional journal manual*. Psychological Assessment Resources.

Deci, E. L., Koestner, R., & Ryan, R. M. (1999). A meta-analytic review of experiments examining the effects of extrinsic rewards on intrinsic motivation. *Psychological Bulletin*, *125*(6), 692–700.

Deci, E. L., & Ryan, R. M. (2012). Self-determination theory in health care and its relations to motivational interviewing: A few comments. *International Journal of Behavioral Nutrition and Physical Activity*. https://doi: 10.1186/1479-5868-9-24

Ellis, A. (1980). Rational-emotive therapy and cognitive behavior therapy: Similarities and differences. *Cognitive Therapy and Research*, *4*(4), 325–340.

Ellis, A. (1991). The revised ABC's of rational-emotive therapy (RET). *Journal of Rational-Emotive Therapy*, *9*(3), 139–172.

Kingdon, D., & Turkington, D. (1994). *Cognitive-behavioural therapy of schizophrenia*. Lawrence A. Earlbaum Associates.

Landa, Y., Silverstein, S., Schwartz, F., & Savitz, A. (2006). Group cognitive behavioral therapy for delusions: Helping patients improve reality testing. *Journal of Contemporary Psychotherapy*, *36*(1), 9–17.

McEvoy, P. M., & Nathan, P. (2007). Perceived costs and benefits of behavioral change: Reconsidering the value of ambivalence for psychotherapy outcomes. *Journal of Clinical Psychology*, *63*(12), 1217–1229.

Miller, W. R., & Rollnick, S. (2012). *Motivational interviewing: Helping people to change* (3rd ed.). Guilford Press.

Ryan, R. M., Lynch, M. F., Vansteenkiste, M., & Deci, E. L. (2010). Motivation and autonomy in counseling, psychotherapy, and behavior change: A look at theory and practice. *The Counseling Psychologist*. https://doi: 10.1177/0011000009359313

Samuel, D. B., Bucher, M. A., & Suzuki, T. (2018). A preliminary probe of personality predicting psychotherapy outcomes: Perspectives from therapists and their clients. *Psychopathology*, *51*(2), 122–129.

Schneider, W., & Klauer, T. (2001). Symptom level, treatment motivation, and the effects of inpatient psychotherapy. *Psychotherapy Research*. https://doi.org/10.1080/713663888

Storch, R. S., & Lane, R. C. (1989). Resistance in mandated psychotherapy: Its function and management. *Journal of Contemporary Psychotherapy*, *19*, 25–38.

Chapter 2

EXPECTATIONS

The expectations a person holds regarding a particular situation influence feelings and contentment with the scenario. If you go to see a movie expecting it to be great and it is not, then you feel disappointed. Hence, it is not just the expectations but the match between expectations and reality, what I refer to as the Expectation-Reality Match (or Mismatch). If you expect the movie to only be okay and it turns out to be better, then you feel good about it because the reality encountered exceeded your expectations. The perception of a gain, consciously or unconsciously, constitutes a cognitive activating appraisal for happiness, with satisfaction and contentment variations. Emotions can be primary or secondary, the former universal including: happiness, interest, sadness, fear, anger, disgust, shame, and surprise (Ekman, 1972, 1994; Ekman & Friesen, 1971; Izard, 1977; Tomkins, 1962, 1963). The research identifying primary emotions transpired with preliterate cultures having limited contact with the outside world, to ensure that they are universal (Boucher & Carlson, 1980; Ekman, 1972). For these primary emotions, there are core circumstances, or what have been referred to as deep structures, expressed in the content of cognitive activating appraisals. The core circumstance for the primary emotions consists of:

Happiness—gain or success (Beck, 1991; Shaver et al., 1987).

Interest—detection of something offering the potential for reward (Izard, 1991).

Sadness—loss (Beck, 1991; Eley & Stevenson, 2000; Finlay-Jones & Brown, 1981).

Fear—threat or danger (Eley & Stevenson, 2000; Finlay-Jones & Brown, 1981; Shaver et al., 1987).

Anger—violation or damage (Rozin et al., 1999; Shaver et al., 1987).

Disgust—contamination, physical or moral (Rozin et al., 1994, 2000).

Shame—a significant social or perhaps moral transgression (Keltner & Buswell, 1997).

Surprise—sudden presence of an unexpected occurrence, either positive or negative (Izard, 1991; Tomkins, 1962).

DOI: 10.4324/b23346-3

Secondary emotions arise either from combinations of primary ones, such as contempt from anger and disgust (Izard, 1994), or points on the primary emotion continuums, as with irritable and annoyed different expressions of anger (Izard, 1994). Given the possibilities for both points on the primary emotion continuums and combinations of primary emotions, the extent of secondary emotions is enormous and many are expressed in psychotherapy. However, for our current focus on expectation-reality matches or mismatches relevant to psychotherapy, we will focus on primary emotions and the various expressions. Hence, when a client perceives that psychotherapy falls below expectations, a loss is perceived with disappointment as a variant of sadness setting in. Conversely, if what is encountered in psychotherapy exceeds expectations, a gain is perceived resulting in happiness, often expressed as satisfaction or contentment. Other primary emotions can be triggered, such as a client perceiving a violation or damage and feeling anger, something reported to me by individuals identifying as homosexual having been exposed to therapy designed to correct this and make them heterosexual. Likewise, I have had clients identifying with being homosexual report that they sensed anti-gay sentiments from a prior therapist, producing a feeling of moral disgust. Emotional information processing is very logical and in many ways straightforward, despite the complexity we often associate with emotions, and it is very helpful for psychotherapists to understand what emotional information processing consists of. It is also very helpful for clients to be aware of it, as when managing sadness and fear, and the amplification of these primary emotions to depression and anxiety, respectively (see the Motivation chapter). In addition, when managing anger and its amplification and expression in the form of aggression, it is crucial to identify and work with perceptions of violation or damage.

As is embodied in the work of Albert Einstein, it is all relative, emotions no exception. How a client sets their expectations, typically unconsciously, greatly influences the match between expectations and encountered reality. A clear example of this relationship and the outcome is with perfectionists who set their expectations at the ceiling. The reality encountered cannot exceed expectations, precluding the possibility of a gain being perceived with happiness and its variants experienced. The best that can be achieved is reality matching expectations, and much more likely, reality falling short of expectations triggering negative emotions, usually consisting of sadness and its variants. This is one reason why during the assessment I usually ask, and always when I sense perfectionism in the client's presentation, "Do you consider yourself to be a perfectionist?" and sometimes the related question, "Have others described you as a perfectionist?" An affirmative answer to these questions informs me that the client will probably set very high expectations for psychotherapy, including their performance and mine. In some instances, a client will only expect perfection from themselves and be more lenient of others, or the reverse scenario, being lenient of themselves and expecting much of others. However, perfectionists commonly view the world in this fashion having high expectations generally. Affirmative responses also inform me that the person is likely self-critical and hence might undermine their progress in psychotherapy. Information pertaining to perfectionism obtained during the assessment and psychotherapy, is rich in consequences for psychotherapy progress. Both the psychotherapist and client can benefit from this information:

Therapist Role

Appreciate that the perfectionistic client is likely to set very high expectations for psychotherapy, thereby setting themselves (and the therapist) up for failure, since the reality encountered will almost certainly fall short of expectations. Addressing the expectation-reality mismatch during the assessment, or early in therapy, is crucial. For example, "I sense that you are a perfectionist and likely have very high expectations for your own performance and maybe that of others. In some instances, perfectionism is required such as manufacturing aircraft brakes according to exact expectations, but human interactions such as psychotherapy do not require it, and can be an opportunity to accept less than perfect outcomes." A statement such as this both helps reset the client's expectations for psychotherapy, such that the reality encountered might exceed expectations, and informs the person that it is okay if they do not perform ideally. Based on my experience, most perfectionistic clients find this reassuring as they and others (or how they perceive others) expect perfection. I often add something to the effect of, "We live in a society that tends to be blame oriented when mistakes occur, but it is far more constructive to accept that mistakes are unavoidable and learn from them." Given that perfectionists naturally drift back to this approach, the message does have to be repeated during psychotherapy when it surfaces. Providing examples of non-perfectionistic perspectives regarding psychotherapy and ones that align with reality is helpful. For example, "Most illnesses are not entirely eliminated, and so some residual depression might persist or return." Assisting the client in resetting their perfectionistic perspective and expectations regarding psychotherapy, including their performance in it, can remove substantial barriers to progress.

Client Role

Accept that you have perfectionistic tendencies (assuming you do) and hence, first, appreciate that you will likely expect too much from psychotherapy, thereby setting yourself up for disappointment. Second, realize that you will expect too much from yourself in psychotherapy and do not have to "perform" to make it work; in contrast, coming to appreciate that mistakes are unavoidable, with psychotherapy a safe setting for learning this, will help make it a very successful experience. Third, appreciate that you might expect too much from your therapist, and like yourself she or he is a person who makes mistakes, no one is perfect. By resetting these expectations, you are more likely to perceive that the reality of the psychotherapy experience exceeds expectations, producing happiness related feelings toward it that motivate. In other words, shifting negative psychotherapy expectations to positive ones will enhance motivation. It is also important to monitor for perfectionistic beliefs pertaining to psychotherapy and raise these with the therapist.

Supporting the relevance of positive expectations pertaining to psychotherapy is research examining the relationship between expectations and outcomes. Constantino et al. (2011) conducted a meta-analysis involving 46 studies with 8,016 clients, examining pre-therapy or early therapy outcome expectations and posttreatment outcomes. They discovered a significant effect of early positive outcome expectations on actual outcomes, and found that these expectations can even influence attendance at the initial session (Constantino et al., 2011), likely because they are linked to hope (Swift et al., 2012). Ongoing positive outcome expectations also impact on outcome, based on a review of 76 studies, finding that clients' persistent expectations for therapeutic gain were related to outcome in most of the studies assessed (Glass et al., 2001). An important component of expectations for therapy consists of reasonable expectations, because if too high, such as becoming a completely different person or no longer experiencing any anxiety, then the reality will fall short of expectations generating disappointment. Dissatisfaction results in failure to progress with psychotherapy (Jung et al., 2013). The generality and specificity of outcome expectations are relevant: based on a review of 35 studies conducted over 25 years, Delsignore and Schnyder (2010) found that global expectancies for therapy were not correlated with clinical improvement, whereas specific expectancies, such as pertaining to the degree of control, were linked to clinical improvement.

To this point we have looked at the role of perfectionism, but will now consider other influences on a client's expectations regarding psychotherapy: the nature of psychotherapy, negative thought biases, and set features of the therapist.

THE NATURE OF PSYCHOTHERAPY

Psychotherapists know about psychotherapy, but prospective clients in some instances do not, or have certain expectations derived from media or other sources. I have a couch in my office, but do not practice traditional psychoanalysis. On several occasions, clients have asked during the assessment, "Should I lie down on the couch." Movies and shows often depict the therapist as a psychoanalyst, although this is changing with more recent versions showing the therapist and client face-to-face. In some instances, I have had clients ask, "Is this CBT (cognitive behavioral therapy)?"

A very interesting aspect of client expectations and the match with the reality of psychotherapy, pertains to the course of therapy. Many things in life work in a linear way, or at least are expected to, such as the longer you work, the more your savings grow. Market volatility, however, clearly indicates that progress is often non-linear, with ups and downs, and fast, slow, and stopped at times. Hayes et al. (2007) looked at this issue for psychotherapy, relying on non-linear dynamical systems theory, with a dynamical system a set of elements that interact and continually evolve over time. There can be critical fluctuations describing substantial challenge to the current steady state of a system, which result in non-linear change with increased variability until the system achieves a new steady state. The researchers indicate that psychotherapy often proceeds in this non-linear fashion, and point to evidence from cognitive behavioral therapy studies of discontinuous change. They explain how the nature of research averaging individual data points can obscure this pattern, making progress with therapy seem more linear, but if individual psychotherapy subjects are examined progress tends to be discontinuous (Hayes et al., 2007). Regarding the relationship between expectations and reality for psychotherapy, this is very important because if a client expects a set amount of progress with each session or number of sessions, and this does not occur, disappointment will set in as the reality has fallen below expectations. The nature of therapy is such that it can take a while for a person to change, as when dealing with abuse issues, a scenario that can even entail worsening symptoms as the person faces the issues, and then suddenly significant progress. In a similar fashion, cognitive therapy takes a while to register on a client, but once the person learns to reframe negative thoughts to more positive variants, the mental health benefits start to flow. An awareness of this reality and adjusting both client and therapist expectations accordingly will foster progress.

At one point in my career I had five male clients over approximately a few years who each worked as management consultants, an occupation that at least then emphasized a linear approach to their effort and the progress of their customers. In therapy, they each took the same approach, such that on a humorous note I began to refer to it as the management consultant perspective on psychotherapy. I carefully explained that psychotherapy commonly does not work in this fashion, and it can take a while for gains to ensue. Four out of the five got it, the light noticeably coming on, and they flexibly altered their expectations for progress, the result being that they progressed well. The fifth would not alter his expectation of linear progress. Given that he had significant abuse issues in his early life, a scenario where mood and functioning can decline before advancing, the persistent expectation for ongoing improvement led to him quitting therapy. Even the interpretation that he might be maintaining that perspective to rationalize not dealing with the painful abuse issues did not sway him. Fortunately, for the other four altering their expectation of linear progress was very helpful for continuing in therapy and advancing.

For therapy to proceed well it is important that client expectations regarding the nature of psychotherapy align with the reality encountered, and both the therapist and client can influence this.

Therapist Role

Client questions like those mentioned regarding psychoanalysis and CBT necessitate an explanation of psychotherapy in general and what type the individual therapist practices. In regard to psychotherapy in general, express something such as, "Psychotherapy is talk therapy for the most part, but there are many different types, such as traditional psychoanalysis where the client lies on the couch and talks freely, and CBT where the focus is on thoughts." There are numerous ways to express the general nature of psychotherapy, although letting the client know that there are variants is always helpful. Appreciating the notion of non-linear change with therapy, it is important to explain that this is how psychotherapy often proceeds, with limited change followed by more rapid change, and not to be disappointed by this occurrence. The next step is to explain the nature of your own practice.

A key issue is whether the type of therapy you provide matches the expectations of the client. If the gap is too great, then therapy best not proceed. For instance, a client Beverly, suffered from Borderline Personality Disorder and depression, with psychotherapy and medication (for depression) stabilizing her functioning. She improved and went several years without any intervention, although for the most part she was unable to work usually remaining on government support. She called me after about five years and indicated that she wanted to resume sessions. However, during the second session she presented that she had been exposed to a different therapy option with an unlicensed therapist and wanted something similar here. This "option" involved more of a personal relationship with equal exchange of information and meeting outside the office. Of course, transference issues enter at this point (see the Transference chapter) and I attempted to work at it from this angle, such as she might have fantasized about a romance or friendship, but this type of interpretation did not work. I also went over how as a client progresses the relationship can seem more equal, and that is normal, but she still insisted on this unique version of psychotherapy. I could not provide it and suggested she seek it elsewhere, with an explanation that licensed therapists do not practice like this.

Therapists can ask the client what they expect from psychotherapy, with a wide range of options feasible, such as the degree of support, symptom change, frequency and length of sessions, the list almost endless. Assess whether what you provide matches the client's expectations, and if not how great is the divide. If too great suggest that the person seeks another form of psychotherapy, but if a narrower gap is revealed, try to bridge it. For example, if the client desires quite a bit of feedback, but your style is not to provide much, attempting to provide more to accommodate the client is reasonable.

Client Role

If uncertain how therapy works, then ask the therapist and/or do some research prior to attending for the assessment. Be aware or wary that there are numerous forms of psychotherapy, and therapists are only familiar with a limited number. As an aside, this is a major practical problem because there are so many forms of therapy with the number increasing yearly, that training institutions, aspiring psychotherapists, funders, and clients are struggling with the situation. In the Impaired States and Processes for Mental Health chapter, I suggest a unified version of psychotherapy, in part due to the overwhelming number of psychotherapy types. Hence, if you look into what psychotherapy involves and are overwhelmed by the options, you are not alone! Instead focus on the general nature of it, and also realize that many psychotherapists practice eclectic psychotherapy, applying techniques from different forms of psychotherapy that are appropriate for a given client at a particular moment. For instance, if a transference issue emerges (see the Transference chapter), then a therapist will (or should) look into this. If you decide that a certain approach to psychotherapy fits best, attempt to find a therapist that provides this. If you are looking for CBT and the therapist is a psychoanalyst, then failure to progress will not be surprising. Appreciate that whatever form of psychotherapy you receive, progress is often non-linear meaning that you might not progress, and might even slip somewhat, before progress kicks in.

NEGATIVE THOUGHT BIAS

People vary in how positive or negative their outlook is, some people perpetually cup half empty maintaining a pessimistic perspective. With depression, a person's outlook usually becomes negative frequently shifting from positive to negative, or more negative in those starting with a negative outlook. How will such a person view psychotherapy? Right, a rhetorical question. Therefore, a client demonstrating a negative outlook, usually evident during the assessment, can be expected to view psychotherapy in a somewhat pessimistic fashion, leading to the perception that their therapy falls below expectations, unless expectations derived from the pessimistic outlook are very low. Interestingly, though, people holding pessimistic outlooks for psychotherapy and other occurrences often still hold quite high expectations, and in some instances these high expectations fuel negativity, since the person realizes that reality is unlikely to match expectations. For various reasons a negative perspective is common in those seeking psychotherapy, and I do not usually encounter a very positive upbeat outlook. Appreciating that pessimism spills over to how psychotherapy is viewed is important for both the therapist and client.

Therapist Role

Asking a client if they have any concerns regarding psychotherapy can help. Negative perspectives will emerge and can be addressed. For example, "No one really gets better, do they?" or "I've heard that people can get more messed up with therapy." Therapy does not have to be "sold" but just explained in a positive and balanced fashion, such as, "Not everyone benefits, but research clearly shows that many people with various problems do improve with psychotherapy." Adding, "If you feel you are not improving please say so and we can see why this is the case." This latter type of statement reassures the client that you are concerned about their progress and will be responsive to feedback. The "we" part emphasizes that it is a relationship for the benefit of the client. The negative thought bias provides a focus for therapy, with a cognitive perspective ideal for addressing the negative thoughts and reframing them in a positive direction.

Client Role

Based on my experience, most clients have a sense of whether they tend to be a cup half full or cup half empty person, and whether their outlook has become more negative. Hence, query yourself regarding these options and realize that if you are prone generally or at this point in time to be negative, then you will probably view psychotherapy in a too negative fashion. Raise concerns with the therapist so they can be addressed, and any negative distortions corrected. Engaging with therapy and focusing on identifying and reframing negative thoughts via a cognitive therapy approach is very helpful.

SET FEATURES OF THE THERAPIST

Every therapist brings fairly or totally set features to the table, as with gender. In some instances, a client will expect a female or male therapist. The scenario where I have seen this most often is females abused by a male (or males) expecting to have a female therapist. In some instances, the circumstances and expectations are milder such as a female client expressing, "I just feel that a female therapist will understand me better." As pertains to this concern, experienced therapists have the capacity to understand a wide range of client issues, and not those restricted to one gender. In a semi-humorous fashion, I have indicated, "A therapist does not have to have schizophrenia, bipolar disorder, depression, anxiety, abuse, eating disorders and the like to understand and work with these issues, and if a therapist was to have them all he or she would not be capable of functioning as a therapist." In addition, the greatest opportunity for progress comes with greater challenge, such as a female who has been abused working with a male therapist, learning that males can be trusted.

Other set features include age and therapist activity level. Despite all the anti-aging options out there, a person cannot hide their approximate age, and for some clients this can be a deal breaker or maker. Some clients will want a therapist approximately their own age, expressing sentiments such as, "A young therapist can't understand what a retiree goes through," and "An older therapist just cannot relate to the culture I'm part of." Often what counts much more than age, though, is compatibility and the connection based on this. For instance, in my case I have a passion for environmental and social justice issues, and young clients with these same concerns tend to bond well to me when they sense this. I am less likely to bond well with developer of my age who is only concerned about making millions of dollars, and disturbed because a lucrative deal fell through.

Activity level is an interesting fairly set feature, because therapists do vary along a continuum of activity level that reflect their personality. Some therapists are very quiet and talk minimally, whereas others are more active and interactive. I tend to lean toward the more active range of the spectrum, and my approach to life is very active with several hobbies and adventure sports combined with travel. If a client appreciates an active therapist, then I will be a better match than a traditional psychoanalyst. Although activity level in therapy can be varied and needs at times to match the client's nature, this is only feasible to a certain extent. If a client is expressing a painful story, even the most active therapist will let the person talk, but overall there will be more talking from an active therapist, and less from a less active therapist.

Therapist and client roles:

Therapist Role

Identify mismatches between client expectations and set features, and then address them right away. If you get the sense that the client is hesitant, mismatch might be a key reason and addressing it is crucial. If a male client expresses that he was hoping for a male therapist because of abuse issues from his mother, then a female therapist can present how the most gain comes from the challenge of a therapist who is the same gender as the abuser. I have encountered this scenario on several occasions with female clients abused by men, and it most often leads to a successful progression. If the client is too fragile and fearful, then suggesting a therapist of the other sex than the abuser might be best. Regarding the age issue, it is best to focus on the connection rather than the age, the value of which most people readily process. In regard to activity level, present what your preferred pattern is and explain why this works. Therapists must be aware that the client might be fearful of therapy in general, and seek a rationalization for not entering into it based on set features. If you sense this might be occurring, express something to the effect of, "It is natural to be hesitant about therapy and people sometimes find reasons to justify not engaging with it." The client might realize that this is what they are doing and appreciate that gender, age, activity level, or another set feature is not the real issue. If the client does not engage with this presentation and other efforts to bridge the gap, it is best to respect their desires and suggest they proceed to another therapist.

Client Role

Consider expectations-match/mismatch as pertains to set features of the therapist, such as gender, age, and activity level. If certain from the outset that you want a therapist with specific criteria, then seek this out rather than react to the therapist encountered. Do not be afraid to ask questions on the phone such as approximate age and activity level (gender will be more evident from the therapist's name and voice). Try to be flexible and appreciate that greater gains often ensue from working with a therapist outside of your comfort zone. For instance, if "straight" and not fond of "gays," working with a therapist who openly identifies with being homosexual might turn out to be the best thing. It generally is not appropriate, at least in my opinion, to ask about the sexual orientation of the therapist.

SUMMARY NOTE

The expectations that clients hold entering into therapy weigh heavily as pertains to psychotherapy progress, and in particular the match or mismatch between client expectations and the reality encountered. Emotional information processing is highly relevant: when reality exceeds expectations, a gain is perceived triggering happiness and variants such as satisfaction; when the reality encountered falls short of expectations, a loss is perceived triggering sadness and variants as with disappointment. A client who experiences satisfaction with therapy is clearly more likely to progress than one who feels disappointed by therapy. Applying the example of a perfectionist, adjusting expectations to a more reasonable level helps ensure that the experience of therapy exceeds expectations. Regarding forms of match/mismatch between expectations and reality, the nature of psychotherapy, negative thought bias, and set features of the therapist are important to consider. Clients have expectations pertaining to the nature of psychotherapy, with an interesting and powerful one consisting of expectations of linear progress. Negative thought bias often results in a client viewing therapy in a negative manner, leading to the perception that the reality encountered falls below expectations. Set features of the therapist, such as gender, age, and activity level, can create a potent mismatch. If both the therapist and client address these sources of match/mismatch between expectations and reality in the ways described, progress with psychotherapy can be enhanced.

REFERENCES

Beck, A. (1991). Cognitive therapy: A 30-year retrospective. *American Psychologist*, 46(4), 368–375.

Boucher, J., & Carlson, G. (1980). Recognition of facial expression in three cultures. *Journal of Cross-Cultural Psychology*, 11, 263–280.

Constantino, M. J., Arnkoff, D. B., Glass, C. R., Armetrano, R. M., & Smith, J. Z. (2011). Expectations. *Journal of Clinical Psychology*, 67(2), 184–192.

Delsignore, A., & Schnyder, U. (2010). Control expectancies as predictors of psychotherapy outcomes: A systematic review. *British Journal of Clinical Psychology*. https://doi.org/10.1348/014466507X226953

Ekman, P. (1972). *Emotions in the human face*. Cambridge University Press.

Ekman, P. (1994). *Antecedent events and emotion metaphors. Nature of emotions*. Oxford University Press.

Ekman, P., & Friesen, W. (1971). Constants across cultures in the face and emotion. *Journal of Personality and Social Psychology, 17*, 124–129.

Eley, T., & Stevenson, J. (2000). Specific life events and chronic experiences differentially associated with depression and anxiety in young twins. *Journal of Abnormal Child Psychology, 28*(4), 383–394.

Finlay-Jones, R., & Brown, G. (1981). Types of stressful life event and the onset of anxiety and depressive disorders. *Psychological Medicine, 11*, 803–815.

Glass, C. R., Arnkoff, D. B., & Shapiro, S. J. (2001). Expectations and preferences. *Psychotherapy: Theory, Research, Practice, Training, 38*(4), 455–461.

Hayes, A. M., Laurenceau, J. P., Feldman, G., Strauss, J. L., & Cardaciotto, L. A. (2007). Change is not always linear: The study of nonlinear and discontinuous patterns of change in psychotherapy. *Clinical Psychology Review, 27*(6), 715–723.

Izard, C. (1977). *Human emotions*. Plenum.

Izard, C. (1991). *The psychology of emotions*. Plenum Press.

Izard, C. (1994). Innate and universal facial expressions: Evidence from developmental and cross-cultural research. *Psychological Bulletin, 115*(2), 288–299.

Jung, S. I., Seralta, F. B., Nunes, M. L., & Elzink, C. L. (2013). Beginning and end of treatment of patients who dropped out of psychoanalytic psychotherapy. *Trends in Psychiatry and Psychotherapy, 35*(3), 181–190.

Keltner, D., & Buswell, B. (1997). Embarrassment: Its distinct form and appeasement functions. *Psychological Bulletin, 122*(3), 250–270.

Rozin, P., Haidt, J., & McCauley, C. (2000). Disgust. In *Handbook of emotions* (2nd ed.). The Guilford Press.

Rozin, P., Lowery, L., & Ebert, R. (1994). Varieties of disgust faces and the structure of disgust. *Journal of Personality and Social Psychology, 66*(5), 870–881.

Rozin, P., Lowery, L., Imada, S., & Haidt, J. (1999). The CAD triad hypothesis: A mapping between three moral emotions (contempt, anger, disgust) and three moral codes (community, autonomy, divinity). *Journal of Personality and Social Psychology, 76*(4), 574–586.

Shaver, P., Schwartz, J., Kirson, D., & O'Connor, C. (1987). Emotion knowledge: Further exploration of a prototype approach. *Journal of Personality and Social Psychology, 52*(6), 1086–1091.

Swift, J. K., Whipple, J. L., & Sandberg, P. (2012). A prediction of initial appointment attendance and initial outcome expectations. *Psychotherapy, 49*(4), 549–556.

Tomkins, S. (1962). *Affect, imagery, consciousness: The positive effects (Vol. 1)*. Springer.

Tomkins, S. (1963). *Affect, imagery, consciousness: The negative effects (Vol. 2)*. Springer.

Chapter 3

PERSONALITY DISORDERS

When psychotherapists think of reasons for why clients fail to progress, one of the first things that typically comes to mind is personality disorders, and certainly Borderline Personality Disorder (BPD). Almost every therapist has had the experience of struggling to make therapy progress with these individuals, only to have it end poorly. Perhaps not surprisingly, psychotherapy outcomes are positively related to the degree of personality organization (more organized better outcomes), based on a systematic review of 18 psychotherapy outcome studies (Koelen et al., 2012). However, progress is definitely possible with disorders of personality, and I have seen substantial gains. Discussions with other therapists support this occurrence, and the outcome is not as bleak as once thought. However, there are significant impediments to progress that can and frequently do arise with these clients. Before looking into the relevant issues, we will take a look at what personality and personality disorders mean.

In general terms, personality can be viewed as enduring and characteristic ways of acting and reacting, a scenario that covers a great deal of potential ground. Attempts to classify personality extends well back into history. In, The Characters, the Greek philosopher Theophrastus listed 30 descriptions organized along one structure, with each character type named and illustrated via examples (in Crocq, 2013). Gerald Heymans set three bipolar dimensions (activity level, emotionality, and primary versus secondary functioning) yielding eight personality types on a cube, consisting of amorphous, sanguine, nervous, choleric, apathetic, phlegmatic, sentimental, and passionate (in Crocq, 2013). Personality was shifted into the psychiatric realm by Emil Kraepelin, who described "psychopathic personalities" of seven types—excitable, irresolute, instinct followers (impulsive), eccentrics, pathological liars and swindlers, enemies of society, and quarrelsome (in Crocq, 2013). Kurt Schneider defined "psychopathic" personality as those individuals who suffer, or cause society to suffer, because of their personality traits, and of great significance, he mentioned that it would be artificial and meaningless to derive clinically relevant abnormal types from exaggerations of normal personality dimensions (in Crocq, 2013).

DOI: 10.4324/b23346-4

Modern depictions of normal personality have emphasized the trait approach, whereby adjectives used to describe personality are listed and subjected to the statistical technique of factor analysis for different populations (Crocq, 2013). Although this research has focused on normal personality a wide range of adjectives, many relevant to personality disorder issues, have been applied. Raymond Cattell's 16-factor system listing bipolar dimensions, referenced by letters to reduce the risk of erroneous interpretations, was the first trait model to be widely recognized (in Crocq, 2013). Then came Cloninger's 7-factor model providing four temperamental dimensions (novelty-seeking, harm avoidance, reward dependence, and persistence) and three dimensions of character (self-directedness, cooperativeness, and self-transcendence) (Cloninger, 1987; Cloninger et al., 1993). The model that has come to dominate is another bipolar one depicting some of the same personality dimensions as Cloninger: the 5-factor Model (FFM) of temperament/personality that has come to be known as the "Big 5" by Costa and McCrae (1992). The five bipolar dimensions consist of: extraversion-introversion, neurotic-emotionally stable, open-closed to experience, agreeable-antagonism, and conscientious-negligence (Costa & McCrae, 1992). In the Motivation chapter, we looked at how openness to experience (as well as conscientiousness) plays a role in motivation for change, thereby linking to psychotherapy progress.

While normal personality depictions were progressing with the fairly objective trait approach, depictions of abnormal personality were rooted or rutted, depending on your perspective, in the categorical and description approach of discrete personality types based on Emil Kraepelin's earlier work, and embodied in the Diagnostic and Statistical Manual of Mental Disorders and International Classification of Diseases (American Psychiatric Association, 2013; First et al., 2002; World Health Organization, 1992, 2022). This categorical approach also relies on a model by Gunderson (1988) providing levels of severity—psychotic type most severe, "self-disorders" including narcissistic, antisocial, and borderline mid-level, and avoidant, dependent, histrionic, obsessive-compulsive closest to normality. Several problems exist with the descriptive discrete model including: excessive co-occurrence of symptoms that should distinguish types, insufficient coverage such that "not otherwise specified" is often the most common diagnosis, arbitrary and shifting boundaries between conditions, inability to manage diverse presentations of a given type, and no real scientific basis (Trull & Durrett, 2005; Widiger & Trull, 2007).

The combination of the less than ideally scientific approach to abnormal personality, and the relatively sound trait approach to normal personality, initiated efforts to depict abnormal personality based on normal personality and more specifically the trait approach. This is a complex area, described in Bowins (2016). However, a key problem is that normal personality dimensions do not directly lead to abnormal personality, even with extreme manifestations, in line with Kurt Schneider's notion that it would be artificial and meaningless to derive clinically relevant abnormal types from exaggerations of normal personality dimensions (in Crocq, 2013). Consider the "Big 5" dimensions of extraversion-introversion, neurotic-emotionally stable, open-closed to experience, agreeable-antagonism, and conscientious-negligence (Costa & McCrae, 1992). Other than for extreme neuroticism, there is no clear abnormal personality depiction, and neuroticism predisposes a person to many mental health disorders, such as anxiety, depression, and somatic issues, not just personality disorders (Bowins, 2010, 2016).

Neuroticism highlights how names for the dimensions do not necessarily capture what is actually occurring. My research suggests that the label neurotic-emotionally stable is incorrect, the more fitting label being reactivity (Bowins, 2010, 2016). I base this assertion, firstly, on how the labels are only that, with Cattell in the 16-factor system applying letters to avoid bias based on labels (in Crocq, 2013). Second, for dimensions of personality to exist in every person, they must have evolved and hence the dimension served an evolutionary function. For example, if the environment offers select areas of valued food sources and predators are not numerous, then high openness to experience is adaptive encouraging exploration, whereas if nutritional needs are satisfied within a limited area and dangerous predators are abundant, then being more closed to experience is most adaptive (Bowins, 2016). Likewise, in a setting where preparation, planning, and perhaps most importantly, perseverance, are required, such as with hunting large prey, being highly conscientious pays off, whereas if resources are easily obtained such preparation, planning, and perseverance only waste resources. Since environments vary, evolution cannot select an ideal level of open-closed to experience and conscientiousness, but instead lays down the dimension providing the capacity for this type of behavior (Bowins, 2016). In the case of "neurotic-emotionally stable" there is no evolutionary logic to it as named, but reactivity is a much different story. In an environment containing dangerous predators, such as crocodiles at watering holes and tigers in the grass, being highly reactive is life saving and hence very adaptive, but in in modern-day industrial society with few such threats, and many social false alarm triggers, lower reactivity is more adaptive. Lower reactivity naturally provides for greater emotional stability. Being highly reactive is so dysfunctional in modern-day society that we, including Costae and McCrae, apply the negative term, "neurotic." Being highly reactive contributes to mental health issues in modern-day industrial society. Hence, if taken as reactivity, instead of neurotic-emotionally stable, the evolutionary function and link to mental illness become more apparent.

Returning to the extension of normal personality to abnormal personality based on the trait approach, there is no solid and comprehensive way to bridge the gap, beyond very specific facets of key personality traits linking to personality disorders (Bowins, 2016). However, the 30 facets of the "Big 5" as an example (see the Personality Factors chapter of the Therapist Influences section) reveal that they could map onto virtually any aspect of human behavior, due to how broad the coverage is. While extending normal personality trait-based approaches to abnormal personality does not work, or is tortuous, viewing personality disorders as extreme and enduring expressions of normal defensive processes does work, is quite seamless, and captures the powerful role of psychological defense mechanisms in personality disorders. In this scenario, these defenses depicting aspects of normal personality become abnormal in an extreme and enduring expression (Bowins, 2010, 2016).

An important note at this point, is that many of the personality disorders focused on have been established through years of clinical experience and research. The ones that appear valid consist of: Avoidant Personality Disorder, Narcissistic Personality Disorder, Dependent Personality Disorder, Obsessive-Compulsive Personality Disorder, Antisocial Personality Disorder, and BPD. Histrionic is an entity rarely encountered aside from traits in my clinical experience and that of other clinicians spoken with, and these traits can easily be explained as a variant of other conditions such as Narcissistic Personality Disorder, Antisocial Personality Disorder, BPD, and Bipolar Disorder. Psychotic personality disorders, referring to Schizotypal, Paranoid, and Schizoid, appear to be part of the psychotic and schizophrenic continuums: "Schizotypal Personality Disorder" being a milder variant of the positive and negative symptoms encountered in schizophrenia, "Paranoid Personality Disorder" involves prominent positive symptoms (delusions) with fewer negative symptoms, and "Schizoid Personality Disorder" more negative symptoms than positive symptoms (Bowins, 2016). However, they do have some defensive aspects as with projection. I proposed the Non-Redundancy Principle (Bowins, 2016), meaning that if a condition best fits into one form of mental illness it should not be duplicated in another form. Psychotic personality disorders best fit into the psychotic and schizophrenic continuums, and so should not be repeated as personality disorders. In a similar fashion, obsessive-compulsive states tend to be ongoing, even though circumstances like depression or anxiety can intensify manifestations, and so best fit under personality disorders (Bowins, 2016), a point we will return to.

Before describing how personality disorders are derived from normal defensive processes, it is worth mentioning that an ongoing problem with psychotherapy for these disorders consists of an us/them mentality. Personality disorder clients are typically viewed as being different, which sets up an in-group/out-group dichotomy hindering progress with psychotherapy. I believe that every therapist has experienced this, with the reaction very intense toward those with BPD. The model of personality disorders based on extreme and enduring expressions of normal defensive processes eliminates or reduces the us/them mentality, because in a milder and more limited fashion everyone has demonstrated the underlying defenses, and it is more difficult to dichotomize when you share what the other person has. Of note, a key notion is to reduce the intensity and persistence of personality disorder behavior into the normal range—normalize. We will now look at how each personality disorder fits with the model of extreme and enduring defensive processes, why impairments to psychotherapy progress transpire, and what can be done to remove or reduce these impediments, emphasizing normalization of the underlying defensive process.

AVOIDANT PERSONALITY DISORDER

The most straightforward personality disorder for understanding how extreme and enduring expressions of normal defenses produce psychopathology, is Avoidant Personality Disorder. Avoidance of threatening and dangerous agents is a normal survival defense. If you see a large predator approaching, you run. Walking up and trying to hug it does not cut it. Less intense but still significant threats are also avoided, such as during the COVID-19 pandemic, many people limited contact with others, thereby reducing the risk of contracting the virus. With Avoidant Personality Disorder, such behavior routinely extents to occurrences that are not objectively threatening and offer the potential for reward. For example, a person might avoid getting a job and/or romance, with these two forms of involvement far removed from the large approaching predator scenario. Dysfunction arises from impaired reinforcement and failure to progress, plus escalating anxiety given how the person never learns that what they fear is not really threatening, and actually offers the possibility of reward. Behavioral inhibition transpires and not behavioral activation associated with good mental health (Alden et al., 2002; Bowins, 2010). Rejecting and isolating experiences often characterize the early life of those with Avoidant Personality Disorder, contributing to a cognitive style of perceiving threats (Alden et al., 2002). Anxiety increases with avoidance, resulting in the perception of more intense threats, leading to more avoidance, and so on and so forth (Meyer, 2002).

Given how the avoidance is so extensive and enduring, psychotherapy for this condition can be a real challenge. What often transpires is that when the client faces the scenario of approaching feared entities and scenarios, they avoid psychotherapy, often rationalizing this decision, such as blaming the therapist for some perceived transgression. This occurrence is not surprising given the engrained nature of their avoidance behavior. Consistent with the dimensional aspect of avoidance behavior, a milder form consists of procrastination that itself can range from mild to intense, the more extreme levels qualifying as Avoidant Personality Disorder. For clinicians, a tip-off that a client might suffer from this personality disorder is the mention of procrastination, as it is a common way that people express avoidance. Despite the challenges of managing more extensive avoidance behavior, including intense procrastination, psychotherapy can progress well with both the therapist and client playing a role.

Therapist Role

The model of personality disorders viewing them as extreme and enduring expressions of normal defensive processes, entails a humanistic approach, and this clearly applies to Avoidant Personality Disorder. Everyone avoids highly threatening agents, and are reluctant to approach less intense threats, such as public speaking for many people. Hence, appreciate that you demonstrate avoidance like the client, but what differs is the intensity and persistent nature of the client's avoidance. A technique that I have found very useful is what I refer to as, "distinguishing the landscape," taking us back to our ancestral hunting-gathering origins, where it was crucial to distinguish real from only perceived threats. For instance, avoiding all moving grass would not help with obtaining food resources, but avoiding grass moving in an unusual manner indicating a stalking predator was life-saving. Help the client identify the landscape of perceived threats, even writing these down. Divide all threats into real and only perceived threats. Since a client with intense avoidance tends to perceive many things as dangerous, another technique is the "100-juror." Have the client image 100 objective jurors deliberating on whether or not the given threat is real. If something in the order of 90% say, yes, then the threat is real. For example, a person driving on a busy street while severely impaired. If the jury is very mixed with maybe 30% thinking there is a real threat, and most not, then it slots into the perceived threat category. If the given threat is real, indicate that it must be avoided. For "perceived" threats divide them into those offering the potential for reward and those that do not. Potential rewards, such as support from a partner or friend, sexual gratification, and financial security might have to be pointed out to the client. Encourage the person to focus on approaching perceived threats offering the potential for reward. Applying the proven behavioral strategy of setting up a hierarchy from least to most threatening is the next step. The client then needs to approach perceived threats offering the potential for reward, working from least to most intense, while reframing the occurrence as being both safe and rewarding. Even the most avoidant client can work with this approach, although some will not progress beyond low level perceived threats despite the reward potential. I have found that antidepressant medication, which is also anti-anxiety medication, can assist clients for whom avoidance is so intensely ingrained that they are effectively in a very deep rut.

A client example will illustrate the application of this technique. I first assessed Jake when he was in his early 40s. For approximately 20 years he maintained the same minimum wage low challenge job, same apartment, no travel, and avoided romance, although he did have friends. Consistent with the notion of non-linear psychotherapy change we encountered in the Expectations chapter, not much progress occurred for quite some time. We identified fears and looked at whether they were real or perceived. He tended to find any change a threat so all seemed real. The 100-juror technique helped him to distinguish the landscape, and with quite a bit of assistance he set up a hierarchy of perceived (not real) threats offering the potential for reward. His first major success in terms of approach behavior consisted of searching for jobs that might be interesting and with better pay, followed by applying, and then accepting one.

This first big change was a catalyst for more rapid approach behavior. Within a relatively short time he started a romance with someone at the new company, traveled with this person, and even did some adventure activities like bungee jumping, most of this, and certainly the adventure activities, inconceivable during the flat progression part of treatment. Adventure activities were not even on the list of things to approach. I have had several other highly avoidant clients follow this path from avoidance to approach and establish it as a pattern. However, I have had several others not progress, in some instances due to reinforcement parameters (see the Reinforcement Parameters chapter). Another helpful strategy is to communicate that 9/10 times the threat is never as bad as imagined.

Client Role

It is important to realize that avoidance of truly threatening agents is a healthy survival defense, but maladaptive when applied to occurrences offering the potential for reward that are not objectively threatening. Engage with the strategies provided for the therapist's role, and work hard on setting up a hierarchy of perceived threats with the potential for reward. Appreciate that progress might be limited at first, but then advance more rapidly as with Jake. Also, accept that in the vast majority of instances what you are perceiving to be dangerous is nowhere near as bad as you think it will be, and in the small minority of instances where it is, approaching the threat and managing it usually plays out best. As the benefits ensue from approaching previously avoided scenarios offering the potential for reward, you will be more motivated and less fearful.

NARCISSISTIC PERSONALITY DISORDER

Both vulnerable and grandiose aspects occur with this personality disorder (Dickinson & Pincus, 2003; Rovik, 2001). The vulnerable side arises from weaknesses and insecurities, while the grandiose side compensates, a counterbalancing of sorts. Fenichel (1945) noted this compensatory relationship, suggesting that excessive achievement striving derives from defective self-esteem. Instead of global self-esteem, more specific weaknesses and insecurities are usually involved, with strengths relied on for compensation. Grandiosity might involve over-control in response to under-controlled aspects, perhaps related to excessive control by parents (Horton & Tritch, 2014). While this might seem like an occurrence restricted to those with Narcissistic Personality Disorder, it is actually a normal and very healthy defense. As an example, if a person is physically uncoordinated but intelligent and scholastic, that individual will rely more on academic achievements for self-confidence and success, whereas someone with the reverse profile will emphasis sporting activities. As these examples show, the defense can be adaptive in terms of success and self-confidence, self-concept, and self-esteem over time.

Compensating for vulnerabilities utilizing strengths is then a natural and healthy defense. Problems arise when the vulnerabilities are profound and the compensation extreme and enduring, first, because the compensation leaves the vulnerabilities in place given that they are never addressed, second, such intense compensation often causes suffering for others, or is very annoying, and third, setbacks repeat from the unbalanced approach and negative reaction from others. Some psychotherapists view vulnerable and grandiose as "types" of Narcissistic Personality Disorder, but I have never encountered one without the other. To simplify information processing, we prefer to clump information and hence see discrete categories, the history of psychiatry rife with this. However, natural entities are organized continuously (Bowins, 2016; Hudziak et al., 2014; Kinsey et al., 1948, 1953). Hudziak et al. (2014) noted that their research group has uncovered many sources of behavioral genetic evidence in support of a dimensional model of mental illness, and express that a categorical (discrete) depiction of psychopathology fails to capture the true nature of behavior and its underlying biology. Many years ago, Kinsey in studying sexual orientation noted both that natural entities are structured continuously and that we have a pronounced tendency to see discreteness (Kinsey et al, 1948; Kinsey et al, 1953). In *Sexual Behavior in the Human Male* (1948), Kinsey and colleagues state, "Males do not represent two discrete populations, heterosexual and homosexual. The world is not divided into sheep and goats. It is a fundamental of taxonomy that nature rarely deals with discrete categories … The living world is a continuum in each and every one of its aspects." They add in *Sexual Behavior in the Human Female* (1953), "It is a characteristic of the human mind that tries to dichotomize in its classification of phenomena … Sexual behavior is either normal or abnormal, socially acceptable or unacceptable, heterosexual or homosexual; and many persons do not want to believe that there are gradations in these matters from one to the other extreme."

From my own research, entities like depression and anxiety are continuous, with extreme variants yielding the impression of discreteness as an emergent property: quantitative variation yields the impression of qualitative variation (Bowins, 2015, 2016). For example, "melancholic depression" appears distinct due to the severe vegetative features, but the extreme range of depression yields these manifestations given the severity (Bowins, 2015, 2016). Likewise, panic attacks an emergent property of severe anxiety, based on the fight/flight/freeze response, that emerges with the supposed "types" of social anxiety, phobias, and generalized worries, when intense (Bowins, 2016). Anxiety is based on the root emotion of fear and circumstances including social, non-social, and thoughts can elicit it with varying severity of expression. It is important to keep this continuous nature of psychological phenomena in mind when we consider mental illness manifestations.

Applying the dimensional model of mental illness to personality disorders based on extreme and enduring expressions of normal defensive processes, fosters a more comprehensive understanding plus strategies to effectively intervene.

Psychotherapy for Narcissistic Personality is often extremely challenging, and in my experience, is more difficult than for BPD, matched for severity level. Frequently, a seemingly benign comment will aggravate the vulnerable side, resulting in anger and/or missed sessions. The client suggests that I do not appreciate his or her skills and accomplishments, instead focusing more on limitations (vulnerabilities), and withdraws from therapy. The grandiose compensatory side often prevents the client from accepting vulnerabilities and effectively partaking in therapy, impeding progress. Ellison et al. (2013) studied 60 severe (pathological) Narcissistic Personality Disorder clients, evaluating both the grandiose and vulnerable sides, finding that the grandiose aspect impaired the use of services and predicted client initiated termination of psychotherapy. Every therapist I have spoken with has experienced this, even though some might not have viewed the person as narcissistic until reflecting on it. Is psychotherapy for this condition hopeless then? Far from it, and there are strategies both the therapist and client can apply.

Therapist Role

Understand that we all compensate for weaknesses and insecurities (vulnerabilities) utilizing strengths, it is just that the vulnerability side is much more profound for these clients, and the compensation relying on strengths too intense and enduring. Frequently, a setback producing depression and/or anxiety will bring the person to therapy, and they rarely identify the vulnerability/overcompensation aspect. I find that both forms of mental illness can be worked on simultaneously, unless depression and anxiety is too severe, in which case it is best to make inroads with such issues first. Frequently, depression and anxiety will obscure the narcissistic aspects, only to be discovered when the presenting issues improve. At this point, some clients feel they have progressed enough and are not interested in addressing "other" issues, only to return to the same therapist or another one when the cycle of profound vulnerabilities, excessive overcompensation, and setbacks arising from the grandiose side ensue. Sadly, I have seen some such individuals continuously replay this cycle over many years.

Even though therapy for Narcissistic Personality Disorder clients is very challenging, I have found that the following approach improves the outcome. First, I express how it is natural to apply strengths to compensate for weaknesses and insecurities with a couple of straightforward examples provided. "If one leg is sore, you put more weight on the other one." "When trying to start a romance a person who is good looking but tongue tied will stand at a party and not say much, whereas a person who is not as good looking but a smooth talker will talk a lot." I have yet to have a client respond that this does not make sense, and nonverbal and/or verbal behavior indicates that it is processed well, in line with how natural the defense is. Then I explain that when the vulnerabilities are more intense, the compensation can be too strong producing setbacks. At this point I indicate how this appears to apply to him or her. Some clients will not accept this, denying vulnerabilities and refusing to view the grandiose behavior as a compensation. As a side note, I never use the term "grandiose" except in the context of mania, where clients often have an inflated sense of importance related to this illness; "overcompensation" is more applicable and easier to digest in the instance of Narcissistic Personality Disorder. For those who are open to the interpretation, real therapy can proceed. Working on both sides of the narcissistic defense is best, having the client identify and address the weaknesses and insecurities, and learn how the overcompensation generates setbacks. Addressing the vulnerabilities often entails reframing perspectives and/or remedying the problem, such as taking steps to complete an academic degree when this limitation fuels self-doubts. Managing the overcompensation involves reducing the intensity of the behavior and finding more moderate substitutes, plus having the person consider how their behavior impacts other people. This combined focus assists the client in healing the vulnerabilities, thereby reducing the need for overcompensation, and shifts the compensatory behavior to more normal limits. A case example will help demonstrate this therapeutic approach.

Roy, a mid-30s businessman, presented with profound depression and anxiety. A major business setback related to a real estate project triggered these manifestations. Initially, I did not see the narcissistic problem, so intense was the depression and anxiety. However, as these problems began to resolve, the role of narcissism became increasingly apparent. His mother was very abusive physically and verbally, continually putting him down, while sparing his more compliant sister. Meanwhile, his father numbed himself with alcohol during the day at business meetings and at night on his own. Consequently, Roy had profound insecurities. Being highly intelligent and with business acumen, he earned a Master of Business Administration degree and embarked on this type of career. His overcompensation and bravado did lead to some real successes, but an equal number of severe failures, and he did not endear himself to many people, contributing to rejection when he asked for assistance with investment concepts. I addressed the vulnerabilities and overcompensation, and although hesitant to accept that his behavior in business was an overcompensation, he at least listened. We worked on how his mother's portrayal of him misrepresented his nature, as he is actually quite thoughtful and empathic. This feedback was very helpful as he just assumed he is a terrible person. He also realized that his father's emotional distancing was not a reflection on him, but simply because his father could not cope with his wife, who insisted at one point that if he tried to leave her she would destroy him financially and take the kids. Defeated, his father numbed himself with alcohol.

Roy's progression based on a more stable foundation with reasonable compensation for the resolving vulnerabilities, was quite amazing. He came up with a very innovative business concept and pursued it in a steady and respectful fashion, leading to a highly successful business. At times a negative comment from an employee or investor aggravated his remaining insecurities, but being aware of what is transpiring he bounced the comments off me to see if there is real merit. So far, his business has persisted well, thereby ending the cycle of setbacks involving overcompensation for insecurities, poor reactions from others, negative mood states, failures, and then a doomed restart.

Client Role

A key here is to be open to the notion that vulnerabilities can and do lead to overcompensation producing setbacks. Everyone has vulnerabilities, even the therapist, and compensating with strengths is a healthy defensive response. The problem occurs when the vulnerabilities are too intense and the overcompensation too extreme and enduring, leading to setbacks that usually replay. Accepting that there is a healthy defensive basis and that you have strengths relied on to compensate helps. Appreciate that the overcompensation does not actually improve the vulnerabilities, but instead locks you into a self-defeating pattern of behavior. Then work with the therapist to strengthen the vulnerabilities and diminish the overcompensation. If you see how the pattern replays over time, with setbacks the end result, there will be more motivation to persevere in therapy even though insecurities can be aggravated. It is best to raise negative feelings that arise when the therapist's comments trigger such a reaction. As vulnerabilities recede, confidence, self-concept, and self-esteem gradually improve, reducing the need for intense compensation, and with the more reasonable compensatory strategies learned, success is much more likely and sustainable.

DEPENDENT PERSONALITY DISORDER

Being a highly social species we rely on others, and even more when stressed. Hence, we are all dependent on others and social support comprises a common defense against emotional distress (Bowins, 2010, 2016). When feeling bad people routinely talk to those they know, and appreciate the other person listening to them and being supportive. However, when dependence escalates to a level where a person cannot function independently, the positive defensive value is compromised. Anxiety intensifies at the slightest threat of not having that support, and without it the person submerges into negative emotions blocking adaptive functioning. The motivation for extreme and enduring dependence is typically anxiety, and by clinging to a receptive person or persons the anxious feelings are reduced, thereby reinforcing the dependent behavior. Certain early life experiences are associated with excessive dependence, such as overprotective, controlling, and authoritarian parenting (Bornstein, 1992; Head et al., 1991).

Most psychotherapists have encountered clients that cling to them, or others in the person's life. Initially, those being clung to can feel uplifted at being valued and helpful, but as the dependency intensifies, annoyance at the intrusiveness sets in. For example, excessive between psychotherapy session phone calls, or emails for therapists who allow this form of interaction. When annoyance sets in the therapist attempts to distance the person through various strategies such as transference interpretation, but this is often not successful. So, what can be done?

Therapist Role

Appreciate that the primary motivation for extreme and enduring dependency is usually anxiety, lessened by social support. The behavioral strategy of having the client set up a hierarchy of stressful independent behaviors from least to most threatening (or stressful) is the first step. The part—have the client—is important because if you the therapist do it all or help too much, then dependency repeats. You can assist but have the client do much of the work. The next step is for the client to work through the list starting with the least stressful. For example, watch another television show in a different room from their partner. The next step might be go out in the garden for a while, or walk around the block on their own. With each accomplishment, a feeling of empowerment usually occurs along with reduced fear, motivating independent behavior for increasingly challenging scenarios. A common problem encountered is for the client to say something to the effect of, "I can't do it as it doesn't feel right." The solution here is actually pivotal to much of psychotherapy: most clients, and even therapists, believe that positive feelings come first and then actions, whereas the reverse sequence is what needs to occur, with the person acting even if not feeling like it and then experiencing the benefits, in this case reduced anxiety and empowerment! I have had this discussion countless times with clients, and those who get it, or are willing to try even if doubtful, almost always report that it works. With effort and time even the most dependent client can learn to become independent, with dependence shifted into the normal range. In some instances, the person will slip back into excessive dependence, and if this occurs consider the possibility of co-dependence, with the person's partner or primary support person threatened by the independence re-establishing the codependent scenario, a problem we will consider further in the Reinforcement Parameters chapter.

Client Role

If you feel fearful at the prospect of independent actions, then you are likely overly dependent. Accept that anxiety underlies this dependence, and the way forward is to become independent in so-called baby steps. To start being independent set up a hierarchy of threatening independent scenarios, with the therapist only providing guidance. Then start progressing through the list from least to most challenging. Give yourself credit for each accomplishment to foster empowerment. Realize that instead of positive feelings preceding actions, act even if not feeling good about it, and let the positive feelings follow from the accomplishment. If your support person is not positive about the changes, then consider the possibility of codependence and discuss it with your therapist. Even though being independent seems too challenging, it is definitely possible, and realize that this does not mean turning into a Clint Eastwood high plains drifter character, as it is normal to seek out people for help and support when stress is pronounced. It just entails having the capacity to function independently and shifting to a normal level of dependence.

OBSESSIVE-COMPULSIVE PERSONALITY DISORDER

Having a way to contain and manage anxiety is very adaptive and defensive. Obsessive-compulsive behavior is that defense, with the obsession representing anxiety and compulsive behavior the containment. Given the discrete nature of psychiatric diagnostic systems (American Psychiatric Association, 2013; World Health Organization, 1992, 2022) the focus is on more intense variants disrupting functioning, but there is a spectrum with the milder variants adaptive. For example, when stressed and worried many people clean or order their environment. The mild compulsive behavior (cleaning or ordering) contains the anxiety. Compulsive ritualistic behavior has been found to maintain tension at a manageable level (Rachman & Hodgson, 1980). Obsessive-compulsive type behavior from an evolutionary perspective, serves the defensive function of minimizing risk by maintaining order (Brune, 2006), or managing various other threats such as contamination or resource depletion (Polimeni et al., 2005). Ninety percent of healthy adults and children demonstrate obsessive-compulsive type behavior, consistent with its common defensive role (Boyer & Lienard, 2006). For example, many people have "nervous habits" such as biting their finger nails that relieve stress in the moment, and increase in frequency and intensity with greater stress. In contrast to milder stress reduced by compulsive behavior, more extreme obsessive-compulsive manifestations lock a person into an endless cycle of intense obsessions and dysfunctional compulsive behavior, such as persistent hand washing or checking.

In some instances, broader fears that are difficult to manage are funneled into more specific fears (obsessions), and contained by compulsive physical or mental behavior. Larry provides an example of this process. In his late 40s, Larry had a successful career in the financial sector, able to purchase a home in a nice area and support his family. Then his world came crashing down from his perspective. He lost his job during a contraction in the market and could not find a suitable one for three years, triggering depression and anxiety. His wife did not "step up" and help by getting a job, but instead criticized him for being "a loser" and not able to support his family and renovate the house. This negativity worsened his mood state and anxiety. Eventually, he took on a job that was less than ideal with very difficult to sell financial products and experienced it as unrewarding. The company eventually sold off its assets and he was unemployed again. Larry experienced worries that were difficult to manage, such as "I've let my family down," I no longer have a career that is viable," "I don't know if I can get back in the game and succeed," "Maybe I am a loser," "How can we fix up the house?" These major worries funneled into obsessions about the house, and compulsive checking behavior temporarily helped to contain the anxiety. Focusing on problems with the house and checking very clear sources of such problems, was much simpler than trying to address the major fears. In therapy, we worked on addressing the more complex fears, and also exposure and response prevention for managing the compulsive behavior and moderating it; he did not want to take medication. Whenever a thought about a house problem emerged he would refrain from inspecting the area, or do so once at most. This technique in combination with addressing the major fears has helped him manage the stress and anxiety.

Larry nicely demonstrates a key issue with obsessive-compulsive behavior and diagnoses. Major diagnostic systems cite obsessive-compulsive behavior as both a primary diagnosis and personality disorder (American Psychiatric Association, 2013; First et al., 2002; World Health Organization, 1992). However, according to the Non-Redundancy Principle (Bowins, 2016), if a given condition best fits into one form of mental illness, it should not be duplicated in another form. So, is it best to cite obsessive-compulsive behavior as a primary disorder or personality disorder? The answer to this depends on how the condition expresses itself. If obsessive-compulsive behavior suddenly manifests like depression with no prior occurrence, then it might qualify as a primary disorder, but if there is a clear milder manifestation that is present before the clinical level expression, then a personality disorder fits best. With the emphasis on discrete entities requiring a certain number of set criteria, the focus has been on obsessive-compulsive behavior as a primary disorder, and only assign it as a personality disorder if the behavior is very persistent. However, in line with 90% of healthy adults and children demonstrating obsessive-compulsive type behavior (Boyer & Lienard, 2006), it is continuously organized, and those with more intense obsessive-compulsive behavior almost always demonstrate milder manifestations when less stressed, although in a categorical diagnostic system framework requiring a certain number of criteria this is missed. Obsessions have been found to vary in how strongly a person adheres to them, indicating a spectrum of intensity (Veale, 2002). Larry acknowledged that he has always been somewhat like this focusing on specific fears, and engaging in compulsive type behavior to manage them. For example, worrying whether he gave a client all the relevant material and checking several times to make sure. When he became depressed and highly stressed, the obsessive-compulsive behavior ramped up enormously. Larry believes that when things do eventually work out for him he will return to milder obsessive foci and compulsive type behavior, which is okay as it actually helps manage fears and contributes to success. Conscientiousness yokes to milder levels of obsessive-compulsive behavior, and I believe that those who are highly conscientious naturally gravitate to an obsessive-compulsive defensive style (Bowins, 2010, 2016). According to the model of personality disorders based on extreme and enduring expressions of defensive processes, normal personality traits predispose a person to certain defensive styles: conscientiousness to Obsessive-Compulsive Personality problems, and closed to experience (harm avoidance) to Avoidant Personality Disorder manifestations, for instance (Bowins, 2010, 2016).

Some readers might suggest that all mental health issues demonstrate some background, such as depression and anxiety, and so why are they not personality disorders? In the case of depression, there can be background factors such as negative thinking, but some people have such thoughts and do not experience depression, while others have mostly positive outlooks that shift to the negative side when the person becomes depressed in response to a significant loss. Sadness-related thoughts are amplified contributing to the onset of depression. Likewise, with anxiety many people tend to be fearful and worry, but do not experience clinical level anxiety manifestations. Threat related thoughts often amplify fears into the realm of anxiety problems. Hence, depression and anxiety are not part of a person's normal personality, unless years of these problems come to characterize their personality, but this is an occurrence following the initial onset of depression and anxiety. Unfortunately, though, with a continuous model of mental illness the lines that we prefer for simplifying information processing do get somewhat blurred.

Obsessive-Compulsive Personality Disorder does raise some intriguing theoretical issues related to diagnosis, but from a practical perspective how can therapists and clients proceed in managing more intense and enduring expressions of such behavior?

Therapist Role

The starting point is working with the notion of obsessive-compulsive behavior as a common defense to contain and manage fears, appreciating that there are a range of expressions with the milder variants normal and healthy. This perspective helps because it bridges the us/them gap, and focuses on normalizing rather than eliminating all traces of obsessive-compulsive behavior, which tends to be impossible and distressing to most clients. The best technique for managing such behavior is exposure and response prevention, having the client contact the obsessive focus behaviorally and/or mentally, and then withhold from acting on it. Anxiety increases at first, but if the person refrains from the compulsive behavior anxiety typically diminishes. Positive self-talk and absorptive-distraction strategies, such as deep breathing and music listening, can be engaged to calm oneself, thereby increasing the chances of the person refraining from the intense compulsive behavior. Clients usually find the notion that milder forms of such behavior are adaptive to be reassuring, and so it is helpful to communicate this. At the same time as exposure and response prevention is engaged, work on the major fears that often drive the more intense and enduring obsessive-compulsive behavior. Assisting the client in dissecting these seemingly intractable fears into manageable components and finding ways to resolve them, does settle the intensified negative emotions, and hence helps to normalize the obsessive-compulsive behavior. Consider a Selective Serotonin Receptor Antagonist (SSRI), that likely works by reducing the anxiety fostering the extreme and enduring manifestations, if exposure and response prevention and psychotherapy do not work adequately.

Client Role

Appreciate first, that obsessions represent fears and compulsive behavior a way of containing the fear, and second, that such behavior is a normal defensive function, problems arising when it becomes extreme and enduring. Conceptualize reducing it to more reasonable normal limits. Also, realize that significant fears and concerns often drive the escalation and work with the therapist to address and resolve them. Engage in exposure and response prevention to manage the extreme obsessive-compulsive behavior, and if this does not work on its own be open to taking an SSRI, with the combination of this type of medication and exposure and response prevention usually very effective.

ANTISOCIAL PERSONALITY DISORDER

This personality disorder is also referred to as psychopathic, dissocial, and sociopath. As discussed, we like to set up discrete categories to simplify information processing, but these are one and the same. "Antisocial" is commonly viewed, even by therapists, as consisting of aggressive criminal activity, but this characterization arises from most studies being conducted with prison populations. Antisocial Personality Disorder at its core consists of enhanced deceit facilitated by dissociation (Bowins, 2010, 2016; Harpending & Sobus, 1987). The evolution of deceit is a fascinating topic, it being present in virtually all species including humans (Harpending & Sobus, 1987). Even young children demonstrate deceit, well before there is any conscious understanding of what their actions entail (Chandler et al., 1989). The reason for why deceit has evolved is that it enables the deceiver to acquire more resources aiding in survival, reproduction, and caring for offspring. If a male bird seeking food for its young makes a quick excursion to impregnate another female, and have that females mate care for the offspring, then his evolutionary fitness is advanced. Likewise, if the female allows the advances of a more robust male, then her offspring will be stronger. If you acquire a resource with a value of 7/10 and return 5/10, you are ahead. However, deceit can be a dangerous game, and violators are penalized and/or ostracized. Hence, refined mechanisms of deceit have evolved.

Antisocial behavior represents an extreme and enduring version of deceit in humans, and a very refined form. Studies of various populations indicate that such a behavior is continuously distributed: prison inmates (Coid & Ullrich, 2010; Marcus et al., 2004), court-ordered substance abusers (Edens et al., 2006; Marcus et al., 2006), non-forensic youth populations (Edens et al., 2011; Murrie et al., 2007), male delinquent youth (Walters, 2014). A study of normal youths by Walters and Ruscio (2013), following 1,708 individuals every 2 years starting at 6 years of age and ending at 14, found evidence for antisocial behavior having a continuous latent structure (Walters & Ruscio, 2013). The continuous organization is consistent with antisocial behavior not just being about violent behavior. Instead, what characterizes antisocial behavior is pronounced deceit (the antisocial part) facilitated by extensive dissociation from the emotional suffering of others, enabling the deceiver to read the emotions of the victim and understand the meaning of the emotion to increase the chances of success, while not being encumbered by remorse and prosocial motivations (see the Emotional Factors chapter in the Therapist Influences section for further information). Factor analyses of the Psychopathy Checklist-Revised, the primary scale for assessing sociopathic behavior, reveals emotional detachment and antisocial behavior as the two main components (Patrick et al., 1994). Both callousness/unemotionality and impulsivity/antisocial behavior are dimensional in convicted offenders (Guay et al., 2007).

Regarding the dissociation component, emotional detachment from, and indifference to, the feelings and welfare of others is a hallmark of the condition (Intrator, 1997). Psychopathic behavior has also been described as a "mask of sanity" in which language and conceptual reasoning are intact, but are dissociated from affect (Patrick et al., 1994). Consider con artists and financial swindlers, able to impress people and gain their trust while emptying their wallets and bank accounts, without any violence at all. To the contrary, antisocial individuals are typically superficially charming and people like them, facilitating deceptions. When violence is present, it is likely an intersection of antisocial behavior and aggressive behavior as an extreme expression of an aggression continuum, and/or brain damage compromising regulation over such behavior (Bowins, 2010, 2016). A fascinating occurrence with antisocial behavior is that it constitutes a seemingly rare instance of frequency dependent selection: when antisocial individuals become too common in a population they are detected and killed off or ostracized (in an evolutionary context often the equivalent), resulting in their number dropping back to a stable equilibrium in the population (Colman & Wilson, 1997). Now that most societies do not kill them off, and in some instance, reward them (think of all those high level financial people who walked away free and clear with millions of dollars from the sub-prime mortgage fiasco of 2008), I suspect that the percentage in the population might be increasing. In this regard, consider the never-ending phone and computer scams.

Hopefully, the discussion of antisocial behavior will alter your perspective helping to explain puzzling behavior, such as why some people seem to consistently deceive, the explanation being that they have a higher capacity on the antisocial and dissociation dimensions of this evolved deceit mechanism. Some readers might still doubt the role of deception, even deceiving themselves about deceit capacity being organized continuously in the population, but consider day-to-day interactions and how low-level deception is adaptive. For example, if your partner or friend does not look great a given day, it is not socially adaptive to say, "You look like crap!" If the person asks, "Do I look good in this outfit that I just bought?" and responding, "It makes you look 20 years older," will not advance your relationship. Excessive honesty does not work and milder deception is normal in social interactions. Another example consists of people pumping up their skill set on resumes instead of being totally honest, often resulting in acquiring a good job over another competitor. However, when the deception is more extreme and enduring much suffering occurs. It might then seem that trying to normalize this behavior is ideal, but unfortunately it does not work, first, due to how antisocial behavior is often highly reinforcing, and second, the evolved nature of both the deceit capacity and dissociation, such that there is no remorse and little if any prosocial motivation. For example, a male who manipulates attractive potential partners into sex by charming them while being detached from the emotional impact, or manipulating clients to enhance financial resources. The evolved deceit strategy is so successful that many antisocial individuals deceive themselves about it, rationalizing their behavior, such as, "If the woman was out in that bar she wanted sex, trust me." "Business is tough and it is survival of the fittest." What if anything can be done then?

Therapist Role

If you encounter a client fitting this description, it is important to realize that therapy might be problematic in that some of these individuals learn from the therapist how to be better manipulators. For example, learning to listen to the other person and show concern in their facial expression, or by supportive comments. An antisocial individual does not empathize given their dissociation from the emotional suffering of others, but can learn to mimic it. Hence, you might be aiding and abetting, despite trying to help. Focusing on other mental health problems and emphasizing consequences ensuing from their actions, is usually the best approach. A client, Tony, presented due to alcohol abuse and depression. The substance abuse was ongoing, but the depression more recent related to being fired from his job at the bank. He discovered that "dead" accounts would often contain small amounts of money, and instead of tracking down the account owners he transferred the money into an account for himself. This went on for several years and was discovered accidently when a customer surfaced and asked about his account. An investigation by the bank led to Tony, and then the dismissal, along with the remaining money being seized. Tony was not remorseful, rationalizing his behavior such as, "Many of those people are dead anyways, so they don't care," "The amounts in each account were nothing so no one really loses," "The bank doesn't pay us well." He did not conceive of himself as antisocial. I focused treatment on the alcohol abuse and depression. One day he attended in obvious distress, due to another scam being discovered and an arrest—checks addressed to other tenants of the apartment building often ended up in his postal box, and he decided to try and cash some. Realizing that community service hours would be more punishment than a very brief jail term and help with sobriety, I wrote a letter to the judge advocating for this. He reported not liking the community service work, and became more aware that there are real consequences to antisocial behavior. Tony is a likable person, and that might have influenced my letter, demonstrating how superficial charm is part of the deception strategy.

Tony's example shows how the best approach is to treat the non-antisocial problems like depression and substance abuse. Also, to make the person aware of their propensity to deceive, even to the point of deceiving themselves about this propensity. From this knowledge, it is prudent to have the client keep in mind that there are consequences that will intensify with repeated offences. Tony only had to remind himself of being fired and those nasty community service hours. As a therapist appreciate and set limits: countless therapists have tried to help and improve antisocial behavior and almost every instance fails. The best that can be reasonably achieved is have the client appreciate the consequences, which is about the only thing that seems to work given how reinforcing the deceit based behavior is.

Client Role

Understand the behavior as a deceit strategy, and see it for what it is without rationalizations. Also, recognize the emotional detachment that facilitates deceptions. Since deceitful behavior is rewarding until caught, at least if there is no remorse, remind yourself ongoing of consequences, which have a way of emerging and intensifying as with Tony. Even though you are predisposed to deceive, those with Antisocial Personality Disorder can consciously resist their urges and lead a relatively ethical life. Resolving addiction issues that lower any restraints on antisocial behavior is also very helpful. Violent antisocial individuals, in contrast to most or almost all white-collar criminals, end up in jail with pronounced consequences.

BORDERLINE PERSONALITY DISORDER

Even though the exact nature of personality disorders is somewhat puzzling, BPD excels in this regard. It is a complex entity and for a full explanation of how it fits with the model of personality disorders based on extreme and enduring expressions of normal defensive processes, see my more extensive coverage in Bowins (2010, 2016). A few key related issues with BPD stand out, the first being trauma during the early years of life. While some researchers such as Gunderson (2009) do not believe that trauma is necessary, other researchers do (Bandelow et al., 2005; Landecker, 1992) aligning with the experience of most clinicians. The crucial element here is, what qualifies as trauma? One option is objective severe trauma, such as sexual abuse. In a study by Bandelow et al. (2005), only 6.1% of their sample did not report any severe traumatic occurrence, compared to 61.5% of the normal control group. Gunderson (2009) referenced this study in asserting that trauma is not necessary, and one of the other two studies referenced, Fossati et al. (1999), only focused on sexual abuse. Hence, even when trauma is restricted to objective severe variants it does appear to be very common in BPD.

The other way of looking at trauma is a subjective perspective, which captures human (and likely animal) nature more accurately (Bowins, 2010, 2016). Trauma is a subjective experience, and what traumatizes one person might not another. For example, a child sent to live with grandparents for a year or two might experience trauma viewing it as abandonment by the parents, while another might see is as an opportunity to have fun with the grandparents. Furthermore, children are more vulnerable to traumatic reactions based on their less developed cognitive structures, global undifferentiated thinking, immature psychological defense mechanisms, and dependence on parental figures (Anguyal, 1965; Levy, 2000). Another crucial issue is the normal personality dimension that we discussed earlier as reactivity, with the negative label of neuroticism. We looked at how normal personality traits favor certain personality disorder expressions, such as conscientiousness Obsessive-Compulsive Personality Disorder and closed to experience Avoidant Personality Disorder. High reactivity (neuroticism) leaves a person much more vulnerable to the impact of objective or subjective trauma, and hence the development of BPD. If clinicians consider their clients with this condition, it does seem that they are highly reactive, and this is due to a high level on this normal personality dimension.

The second key feature of BPD is emotional dysregulation, which in the context of high reactivity alone even makes sense. Examining electronic diary entries of those with BPD and normal subjects, Ebner-Priemer et al. (2015) found that those with BPD had a more negative emotional baseline and greater variability. Comparing emotional regulation dysfunction, problematic relations, and nonintegrated self, Cheavens et al. (2012) discovered that the former had the strongest relationship to BPD symptoms. Emotional regulation mediates the relationship between BPD symptom severity and interpersonal dysfunction, based on results from an adult study (Herr et al., 2013). Volatility of emotions is extremely common in BPD, something every therapist working with these individuals has experienced. Gratz and Roemer (2004) have identified components of emotional dysregulation: lack of awareness of emotional responses, lack of clarity of emotional responses, non-acceptance of emotional responses, limited access to emotion regulation strategies perceived as effective, difficulties controlling impulses when experiencing negative emotions, and difficulties engaging in goal-directed behaviors when experiencing negative emotions. BPD clients typically experience impairments with several of these components, and significant improvement in psychotherapy entails awareness of emotional responses, clarity of emotional responses, acceptance of emotional responses, access to emotion regulation strategies perceived as effective, controlling impulses when experiencing negative emotions, and engaging in goal-directed behaviors when experiencing negative emotions. High emotion regulation capacities provide for solid emotional intelligence. Links et al. (2017) found that enhancing emotion regulation is an important mechanism of positive change for BPD clients, based on a review of 16 studies.

More significant than high reactivity for emotional dysregulation is the third key feature of BPD, reliance on immature psychological defense mechanisms including acting out, splitting, idealization-devaluation, and projective identification (Bond & Perry, 2004; Bond et al., 1994; Landecker, 1992; Perry, 2001; Van Wijk-Herbrink et al., 2011). Maladaptive and image distorting immature defense mechanisms characterize BPD (Kernberg, 1976). Bond et al. (1994) suggest that intense and long-term use of immature defenses contributes to the development of BPD symptoms. Progress with therapy entails a shift from immature defenses to mature ones, such as sublimation, suppression, altruism, and humor (Bond & Perry, 2004; Perry, 2001; Van Wijk-Herbrink et al., 2011). My clinical experience supports this, with the presence and reliance on immature defense mechanisms characterizing their dysfunctional behavior, and real progress occurring when these defenses are replaced with mature ones. A major reason why these immature defenses are so dysfunctional, in at least the later adolescent and adult age range, is that they foster emotional dysregulation. Acting out leads to unfiltered expression of emotions, usually negative but this can alternate with excessive displays of warmth and excitement. Splitting and idealization-devaluation produce intense shifts in emotions, between people in the case of splitting and for one person with idealization-devaluation, usually involving the therapist in both instances. With projective identification, the client elicits the negative emotion, usually anger, in the therapist to identify with the emotion, at which point the client calms and the therapist reacts, sometimes triggering a negative response in the client. Contrast this emotional rollercoaster induced by immature defenses to mature defense mechanism: sublimation transforms negative energy into constructive foci and pursuits, suppression suspends a negative emotion in the moment when its expression is maladaptive, altruism encourages the person to treat others as they wish to be treated, and humor eases tension by placing a lighter spin on events. In essence, immature psychological defense mechanisms foster emotional dysregulation while mature defenses favor emotional regulation.

An important question is what causes those with BPD to utilize immature defense mechanisms? The answer lies in the impact of trauma, objective and subjective, on defense mechanisms, and particularly when a person is highly reactive by nature. When a person experiences trauma defense mechanisms are employed to cope, and given the lasting impact of trauma they are expressed in an ongoing fashion, thereby coming to characterize personality. If a person has reached adulthood and developed mature defenses, then these sophisticated defenses are expressed to cope, an occurrence that will help resolve or minimize the traumatic reaction. However, during childhood and adolescence when immature defenses are the norm, defenses such as acting out, splitting, idealization-devaluation, and projective identification are applied to cope to such an extent that they come to characterize the individual, and due to their limitations perpetuate the suffering (Bowins, 2010, 2016; Cramer & Block, 1998; Finzi-Dottan & Karu, 2006). In other words, psychological defense mechanism development becomes frozen with trauma, and I also believe that the regulation of defense mechanisms, referring to activation of the defense, monitoring of its impact, and deactivation, is also frozen at an immature level (Bowins, 2010, 2016).

The individual unconsciously applies immature defenses mechanisms ongoing and struggles to regulate their use, resulting in emotional dysregulation, volatile relationships generating more stress, coped with by the use of immature defenses, and so on and so forth. The trigger for this endless negative cycle is trauma prior to adulthood before mature defenses develop. From the perspective of the therapist and client, there are many viable interventions and entire books have been written about therapy for BPD clients. I will not try and cover the extent of possible interventions, but focus on interventions derived from the model of abnormal personality based on extreme and enduring expressions of normal defensive processes, which in the case of BPD refers to, first, how we all have utilized immature defenses during childhood and adolescence, and second, defining normal as the utilization of mature defense during adulthood, with a focus on normalizing the BPD client in terms of adopting age-appropriate defenses.

Therapist Role

A frequent occurrence in therapy is therapists reacting to the BPD client in regard to their emotional dysregulation and the behavior following from it, such as outbursts of anger, aggression, sadness, and fear. By focusing on defense mechanisms and emotional dysregulation, therapists regain a sense of proactive control. Given that progress in therapy aligns with the shift from immature to mature defense, and failure to progress entails no maturation of these defenses (Bond & Perry, 2004; Bond et al., 1994; Kernberg, 1976; Landecker, 1992; Perry, 2001; Van Wijk-Herbrink et al., 2011), I attempt to fast forward the process by directly fostering the development of mature defenses. Unlike immature and intermediate level defenses, mature ones can be consciously fostered such as by encouraging a humorous outlook and sublimating negativity into positive foci. A starting point is identifying the immature (and any more mature) defenses the BPD client utilizes. Obviously, this entails an understanding of classical psychological defense mechanisms and the range from immature to mature. Discuss immature defenses noted, based on client-therapist interactions and reported relationships outside of therapy, demonstrating how their use generates emotional instability. For example, "When I mentioned I will be away for a week, you compared me negatively to your prior therapist who never went on vacation, making you distressed at the prospect of being abandoned." This statement describes splitting and the resulting emotional dysregulation. Likewise, with anger expressed at a perceived violation, "You thought that I did something to offend you and then just expressed this without considering if it's true or not." This statement captures acting out and how emotional regulation over anger suffered as a result. Projective identification is trickier to work with but a therapist can approach it by saying, "I am finding myself getting angry, something that is not common in sessions, and I believe it is because I am feeling and expressing your anger." It is helpful to go over how we all have used these defenses, but with traumatic events earlier in life they are overused.

The next step is to discuss mature defense mechanisms and demonstrate how they foster improved emotional stability compared to immature ones. Examples taken from sessions and events outside of therapy can be used. Emphasis how adaptive it is to shift to these more mature defenses, and how with frequent application they will replace the less mature ones. Any expression of immature defenses is to be addressed. With this focus the all-important transition from immature to mature psychological defenses, and resulting shift from emotional dysregulation to regulation, can be accelerated, hopefully at least. If the BPD client shows any mature defensive capacity foster more of this. For example, I recall one young female client who had a great sense of humor, at least when in a positive mood, and applying it helped smooth out stresses in therapy, plus motivated her to adopt other mature defenses. Regarding psychological defense mechanism regulation (as well as emotion regulation), therapists typically function at a mature level, evidenced in how they manage interactions with the BPD client, setting a model for the client to internalize. Additional important issues, such as the impact of trauma, bonding and the therapeutic alliance, and transference and countertransference, also applicable to patients not having BPD, will be covered in other chapters. A crucial issue in managing BPD is the client's level of functioning, and certainly in terms of emotional regulation. Based on my experience, and I have tried, very low functioning individuals do not do well in one-to-one therapy, and group therapy is best to help stabilize their functioning, such that they can tolerate the therapeutic alliance. I know a female therapist who tried to run a practice with mostly low functioning BPD individuals and gave up after about two years as she was going "insane" and it was either change the nature of her practice or quit. Hence do not view yourself as Superwoman of Superman, or be a martyr!

Client Role

If your functioning is very limited accept that one-to-one therapy is not the starting point, and instead group therapy designed to foster emotional and behavioral regulation is most optimal, at least to start. Regardless of the therapeutic setting appreciate that emotional dysregulation is a key aspect of the difficulties experienced, and this largely arises from the overuse of immature, less adaptive psychological defense mechanisms. These defenses are almost certain to generate emotional instability in adults. On the other hand, mature defenses, such as those mentioned, foster emotional and relationship stability. Actively work on replacing immature defenses with mature ones, by practicing in therapy and out of therapy. Every instance of progress in therapy for BPD I have seen entailed shifting from immature to mature defenses, with research backing this up. Conversely, failure to progress involves the retention of immature defenses with the resulting emotional volatility. Other aspects of psychological functioning, such as trust and trauma impacts, have to be worked on, but these will be assisted by the application of mature defenses.

SUMMARY NOTE

Having a personality disorder does work against progress in therapy, but yet tremendous progress can be made with the right understanding of these conditions and approach. The model of personality disorders based on extreme and enduring expressions of normal and healthy defensive processes, does fit well with the nature of these problems, and resolves the difficulties encountered in attempting to extend normal trait-based personality descriptions to abnormal personality. Instead, normal personality traits predispose a person to certain defensive styles that can morph into a personality disorder under the right, or depending on your perspective, wrong, circumstances. For example, closed to experience for Avoidant Personality Disorder, conscientiousness for Obsessive-Compulsive Personality Disorder, and high reactivity (neuroticism) to BPD. Focusing on normalizing the underlying defensive process in the ways described for each personality disorder will assist with therapy progress. As a therapist, realize that even with optimal performance progress can be limited, consistent with lower levels of personality organization resulting in worse psychotherapy outcomes (Koelen et al., 2012). Instead of being self-critical, learn from the experience and apply this knowledge to future therapy sessions for personality disorder clients!

REFERENCES

Alden, L. E., Laposa, J. M., Taylor, C. T., & Ryder, A. G. (2002). Avoidant personality disorder: Current status and future directions. *Journal of Personality Disorders*, *16*(1), 1–29.

American Psychiatric Association. (2013). *Diagnostic & statistical manual 5*. American Psychiatric Publishing Inc.

Anguyal, A. (1965). *Neurosis and treatment: A holistic theory*. Wiley.

Bandelow, B., Krause, J., Wedekind, D., Broocks, A., Hajak, E., & Ruther, E. (2005). Early traumatic life events, parental attitudes, family history, and birth risk factors in patients with borderline personality disorder and healthy controls. *Psychiatry Research*, *134*, 169–179.

Bond, M., Paris, J., & Zweig-Frank, H. (1994). The defense style questionnaire in borderline personality disorder. *Journal of Personality Disorder, 8,* 28–31.

Bond, M., & Perry, J. C. (2004). Long-term changes in defense styles with psychodynamic psychotherapy for depressive, anxiety, and personality disorders. *American Journal of Psychiatry, 161*(9), 1665–1671.

Bornstein, R. F. (1992). The dependent personality: Development, social, and clinical perspectives. *Psychological Bulletin, 112*(1), 3–23.

Bowins, B. E. (2010). Personality disorders: A dimensional defense mechanism approach. *American Journal of Psychotherapy, 64*(2), 153–169.

Bowins, B. E. (2015). Depression: Discrete or continuous? *Psychopathology, 48*(2), 69–78.

Bowins, B. E. (2016). *Mental illness defined: Continuums, regulation, and defense.* Routledge.

Boyer, P., & Lienard, P. (2006). Why ritualized behavior? Precaution systems and action parsing in developmental, pathological and cultural rituals. *Behavioural and Brain Science, 29,* 595–613.

Brune, M. (2006). The evolutionary psychology of obsessive-compulsive disorder. *Perspectives in Biology and Medicine, 49*(3), 317–329.

Chandler, M., Fritz, A., & Hala, S. (1989). Small-scale deceit: Deception as a marker of two, three, and four-year-olds early theories of mind. *Child Development, 60,* 1263–1277.

Cheavens, J. S., Strunk, D. R., & Chriki, L. (2012). A comparison of three theoretically important constructs: What accounts for symptoms of borderline personality disorder? *Journal of Clinical Psychology, 68*(4), 477–486.

Cloninger, C. R. (1987). A systematic method for clinical description and classification of personality variants. *Archives of General Psychiatry, 44,* 573–588.

Cloninger, C. R., Svrakic, D. M., & Przybeck, T. R. (1993). A psychobiological model of temperament and character. *Archives of General Psychiatry, 50,* 975–990.

Coid, J., & Ullrich, S. (2010). Antisocial personality disorder is on a continuum with psychopathy. *Comprehensive Psychiatry, 51*(4), 426–433.

Colman, A. M., & Wilson, J. C. (1997). Antisocial personality disorder: An evolutionary game theory analysis. *Legal and Criminological Psychology, 2*(1), 23–34.

Costa, P. T., & McCrae, R. R. (1992). *Revised NEO personality (NEO-PI-R) and NEO five factor inventory (NEO-FFI) professional journal manual.* Psychological Assessment Resources.

Cramer, P., & Block, J. (1998). Preschool antecedents of defense mechanism use in young adults: A longitudinal study. *Journal of Personality & Social Psychology, 74,* 159–169.

Crocq, M. A. (2013). Milestones in the history of personality disorders. *Dialogues Clinical Neuroscience, 15*(2), 147–153.

Dickinson, K. A., & Pincus, A. L. (2003). Interpersonal analysis of grandiose and vulnerable narcissism. *Journal of Personality Disorders, 17,* 188–207.

Ebner-Priemer, U. W., Houben, M., Santangelo, P., Kleindienst, N., Tuerlinckx, F., Oravecz, Z., et al. (2015). Unraveling affective dysregulation in borderline personality disorder: A theoretical model and empirical evidence. *Journal of Abnormal Psychology, 124*(1), 186–198.

Edens, J. F., Marcus, D. K., Lilienfeld, S. O., & Poythress, N. G. Jr. (2006). Psychopathic, not psychopath: Taxometric evidence for the dimensional structure of psychopathy. *Journal of Abnormal Psychology, 115*(1), 131–144.

Edens, J. F., Marcus, D. K., & Vaughn, M. G. (2011). Exploring the taxometric status of psychopathy among youthful offenders: Is there a juvenile psychopath taxon? *Law & Human Behavior, 35*(1), 13–24.

Ellison, W. D., Levy, K. N., Cain, N. M., Ansell, E. B., & Pincus, A. L. (2013). The impact of pathological narcissism on psychotherapy utilization, initial symptom severity, and early-treatment symptom change: A naturalistic investigation. *Journal of Personality Assessment, 95*(3), 291–300.

Fenichel, O. (1945). *The psychoanalytic theory of neurosis.* Norton & Company.

Finzi-Dottan, R., & Karu, T. (2006). From emotional abuse in childhood to psychopathology in adulthood: A path mediated by immature defense mechanisms and self-esteem. *The Journal of Nervous and Mental Disease, 194*(8), 616–620.

First, M. B., Frances, A., & Pincus, H. A. (2002). *DSM-IV-TR handbook of differential diagnosis.* American Psychiatric Publishing.

Fossati, A., Madeddu, F., & Maffei, C. (1999). Borderline personality disorder and childhood sexual abuse. *Journal of Personality Disorders, 13*(3), 268–280.

Gratz, K. L., & Roemer, L. (2004). Multidimensional assessment of emotion regulation and dysregulation: Development, factor structure, and initial validation of the difficulties in emotion regulation scale. *Journal of Psychopathology and Behavioral Assessment, 26,* 41–54.

Guay, J. P., Ruscio, J., Knight, R. A., & Hare, R. D. (2007). A taxometric analysis of the latent structure of psychopathy: Evidence for dimensionality. *Journal of Abnormal Psychology, 116*(4), 701–716.

Gunderson, J. G. (1988). Personality disorders. In A. M. Nicholi (Ed.), *The new Harvard guide to psychiatry* (pp. 337–357). Harvard University Press.

Gunderson, J. G. (2009). Borderline personality disorder: Ontogeny of a diagnosis. *American Journal of Psychiatry, 166*(5), 530–539.

Harpending, H., & Sobus, J. (1987). Sociopathy as an adaptation. *Ethology and Sociobiology, 8,* 63S–72S.

Head, S. B., Baker, J. D., & Williamson, D. A. (1991). Family environment characteristics and dependent personality disorder. *Journal of Personality Disorders, 5*(3), 256–263.

Herr, N. R., Rosenthal, M. Z., Geiger, P. J., & Erikson, K. (2013). Difficulties with emotional regulation mediate the relationship between borderline personality disorder symptom severity and interpersonal problems. *Personality & Mental Health, 7*(3), 191–202.

Horton, R. S., & Tritch, T. (2014). Clarifying the links between grandiose narcissism and parenting. *Journal of Psychology, 148*(2), 133–143.

Hudziak, J. J., Albaugh, M. D., Ducharme, S., Karama, S., Spottswood, M., Crehan, E., et al. (2014). Cortical thickening maturation and duration of music training: Health-promoting activities shape brain development. *Journal of the American Academy of Child and Adolescent Psychiatry, 53*(11), 1153–1161.

Intrator, J. (1997). A brain imaging (single photon emission computerized tomography) study of semantic and affective processing in psychopaths. *Biological Psychiatry, 42,* 96–103.

Kernberg, O. F. (1976). *Borderline conditions and pathological narcissism.* Jason Aronson.

Kinsey, A. C., Pomeroy, W. B., & Martin, C. E. (1948). *Sexual behavior in the human male.* W.B. Saunders.

Kinsey, A. C., Pomeroy, W. B., Martin, C. E., & Gebhard, P. H. (1953). *Sexual behavior in the human female.* W.B. Saunders.

Koelen, J. A., Luyten, P., Eurelings-Bontekoe, L. H., Diguer, L., Vermote, R., Lowyck, et al. (2012). The impact of level of personality organization on treatment response: A systematic review. *Psychiatry, 75*(4), 355–374.

Landecker, H. (1992). The role of childhood sexual trauma in the etiology of borderline personality disorder: Considerations for diagnosis and treatment. *Psychotherapy, 29*(2), 234–242.

Levy, M. (2000). A conceptualization of the repetition compulsion. *Psychiatry, 63,* 45–53.

Links, P. S., Shah, R., & Eynan, R. (2017). Psychotherapy for borderline personality disorder: Progress and remaining challenges. *Current Psychiatry Report, 19*(3), https://doi.org/10.1007/s11920-017-0766-x

Marcus, D. K., John, S. L., & Edens, J. F. (2004). A taxometric analysis of psychopathic personality. *Journal of Abnormal Psychology*, *113*(4), 626–635.

Marcus, D. K., Lilienfeld, S. O., Edens, J. F., & Poythress, N. G. (2006). Is antisocial personality disorder continuous or categorical? A taxometric analysis. *Psychological Medicine*, *36*(11), 1571–1581.

Meyer, B. (2002). Personality and mood correlates of avoidant personality disorder. *Journal of Personality Disorders*, *16*(2), 174–188.

Murrie, D. C., Marcus, D. K., Douglas, K. S., Lee, Z., Salekin, R. T., & Vincent, G. (2007). Youth with psychopathy features are not a discrete class: A taxometric analysis. *Journal of Child Psychology & Psychiatry*, *48*(7), 714–723.

Patrick, C., Cuthbert, B., & Lang, P. (1994). Emotion in the criminal psychopath: Fear image processing. *Journal of Abnormal Psychology*, *103*(3), 523–534.

Perry, C. (2001). A pilot study of defenses in adults with personality disorders entering psychotherapy. *The Journal of Nervous and Mental Disease*, *189*, 651–660.

Polimeni, J., Reiss, J. P., & Sareen, J. (2005). Could obsessive-compulsive disorder have originated as a group-selected adaptive trait in traditional societies? *Medical Hypothesis*, *65*, 655–664.

Rachman, S., & Hodgson, R. (1980). *Obsessions and compulsions*. Prentice-Hall.

Rovik, J. O. (2001). Overt and covert narcissism: Turning points and mutative elements in two psychotherapies. *British Journal of Psychotherapy*, *17*, 435–447.

Trull, T. J., & Durrett, C. A. (2005). Categorical and dimensional models of personality disorder. *Annual Review of Clinical Psychology*, *1*, 355–380.

Van Wijk-Herbrink, M., Andrea, H., & Verheul, R. (2011). Cognitive coping and defense styles in patients with personality disorders. *Journal of Personality Disorders*, *25*(5), 634–644.

Veale, D. (2002). Over-valued ideas: A conceptual analysis. *Behavioural Research & Therapy*, *40*(4), 383–400.

Walters, G. D. (2014). The latent structure of psychopathy in male adjudicated delinquents: A cross-domain taxometric analysis. *Personality Disorders*, *5*(4), 348–355.

Walters, G. D., & Ruscio, J. (2013). Trajectories of youthful antisocial behavior: Categories or continua? *Journal of Abnormal Child Psychology*, *41*(4), 653–666.

Widiger, T. A., & Trull, T. J. (2007). Plate tectonics in the classification of personality disorder: Shifting to a dimensional model. *American Psychologist*, *62*(2), 71–83.

World Health Organization. (1992). *The ICD-10 classification of mental and behavioral disorders: Clinical descriptions and diagnostic guidelines*. World Health Organization.

World Health Organization. (2022). *The ICD-10 classification of mental and behavioral disorders: Clinical descriptions and diagnostic guidelines*. World Health Organization.

Chapter 4

REINFORCEMENT PARAMETERS

Reinforcement strengthens a given behavior, increasing its frequency. Positive reinforcement occurs when a behavior results in a positive outcome, such as you approach your partner and get a warm hug, or purchase an item you really like. Negative reinforcement refers to the elimination or reduction of an adverse experience. A classic example being children whining when they want something, and the purchase of that something removing the adversity of the whining. In a similar fashion, your furnace dies on a cold night creating an adverse experience, eliminated by having the furnace technician fix it. When most people think of reinforcement they usually only consider the positive variant, but negative reinforcement can be potent. Think of the relief felt when a whining child ceases the behavior with a purchase, or elimination of pain at the removal of a sliver. The same occurrence can involve both positive and negative reinforcement, with the event introducing something rewarding and also relieving distress. For instance, you need your car to get around but it is always breaking down, creating the adverse feeling of apprehension about being stranded, so you purchase a new car that you like (positive reinforcement), and feel enormous relief not having to worry about a breakdown and getting stranded (negative reinforcement). In contrast to reinforcement, punishment reduces the frequency of a behavior, such as spanking a child, or prison when convicted of a significant crime. A problem with punishment, as might come to mind at the prison example at least, is that it has variable effects, sometimes reducing the frequency of a behavior, and in other instances leading to more secrecy and manipulation, as with prison inmates learning to become more effective criminals, and children hiding the behavior that got them into trouble.

Reinforcement impacts enormously on all aspects of day-to-day life, and psychotherapy is no exception, including progression. However, other than for behavioral therapists, reinforcement is rarely focused on. My favorite example of reinforcement impacting on psychotherapy progress is a personal anecdote. Several years ago, I happened to have five young clients who all fit the same approximate bill, anxiety and some depression issues, with each person on welfare. The mood symptoms and welfare reinforced each other in that the anxiety

DOI: 10.4324/b23346-5

and depression intensified avoidance of work, and the limited financial standing and status of being on welfare strengthened the mood issues. As an aside, when this type of process occurs therapists often refer to "cycles" or "loops," but "mutual reinforcement" is a more appropriate term, as both sides of the equation are strengthened increasing their frequency. For instance, with negative thoughts and negative emotions, the thoughts generate negative emotions such as sadness, which creates an emotional climate conducive to further negative thoughts, and so on and so forth, the thoughts and emotional states mutually reinforcing each other.

Getting back to my five clients example, I attempted to get each of these individuals to face their fears pertaining to work, and advance in their lives, thinking that the empowerment and self-confidence gains would lessen symptoms of anxiety and depression, a basically correct assumption. Antidepressant medication was used for three of them to lessen adverse mood states and help them face the challenge, but nothing worked. It turned out that I missed a potent source of reinforcement! At this point in time Ontario had a more socialist government, the New Democratic Party, and hence very generous welfare payments were made. Relative to what I would consider a decent income, the payments seemed paltry, but were enough that these five clients could afford reasonable apartments (at that time housing costs in Toronto were very low), purchase food, and have some entertainment money. In the language of reinforcement, their avoidant lifestyle and not progressing in terms of employment was being strongly reinforced. During the next election, the Progressive Conservative Party was voted in, with Premier Mike Harris at the helm. His platform entailed minimal government support and welfare payments were high on his list of things to cut. Suddenly, these payments dropped about 30%, and almost equally fast, all five of my clients were working! Two main possibilities consist of, first, Premier Harris was a much better therapist, and, second, he altered the reinforcement parameters such that a job was the best option for these five clients. Although I could be accused of taking a self-enhancing stance, I believe that it was the second scenario, particularly considering that the Premier had no psychotherapy experience I am aware of. The reduced welfare payments made it realistically impossible for these clients to lead a comfortable life, thereby creating substantial adversity, reduced by getting a job that paid more (negative reinforcement). As I predicted, despite some initial fears all five clients progressed in terms of less anxiety and depression, and improved self-confidence and empowerment. That experience was a powerful one for me as a psychotherapist, pertaining to how potent reinforcement parameters can be for progress, or failure to progress, in therapy, and how all sources of reinforcement need to be considered. The example also highlights how some people will take the less stressful path even to their own long range detriment, and how social justice strategies need factor in reinforcement effects.

Hopefully, my personal anecdote and the reasons for why positive and negative reinforcement is so potent, will convince you of the importance of reinforcement parameters. We will now look at various manifestations focusing on how failure to progress in psychotherapy can be due to reinforcement effects. While the divisions are somewhat artificial and should not be viewed as clear types, I will divide them into structural, psychopathology, and codependence. It is important to note that reinforcement can increase success in therapy, as for example, a client's partner greatly appreciating changes and encouraging the person to continue, or the client feeling much better, but the focus here is on impediments to progress.

STRUCTURAL

By the term "structural" I am referring to reinforcement parameters independent of mental illness manifestations and personal issues. My five-client example above qualifies, as despite somewhat individual forms of psychopathology and characteristics, each was potently reinforced by the structure of welfare payments relative to the lifestyle afforded by those payments. Another very common structural reinforcement parameter pertains to payments for psychotherapy. In most settings around the world, the government does not cover payments for psychotherapy, or only partially. In Ontario and most of Canada, the provincial governments do cover payments, at least so far. If the government system does not pay, where does the money come from? In many instances the answer is insurance, but these plans only cover so many sessions. A limited number of sessions is inadequate for complex issues and can really only address one item, such as depression or anxiety, with packaged short-term interventions. Funding beyond these very limited amounts, then involves payments by the client. If the person is independently wealthy or at least well off, then no problem, but since very few people have this degree of financial security choices have to be made. If the choice is between psychotherapy and food, shelter, medicine, needs of children, some relief from the tedium of day-to-day life, and the like, then the reinforcement parameters usually do not favor psychotherapy, or sticking with it beyond a very limited number of sessions. Food, shelter, medicine, needs of children, and some relief from the tedium of day-to-day life offer both positive reinforcement and negative reinforcement, such as food being rewarding and relieving hunger. Psychotherapy, meanwhile, offers less salient reinforcement such as better mood states and less emotional suffering. Given these reinforcement parameters most people will not opt for psychotherapy. Hence, the importance of highly affordable psychotherapy. I have had clients from other parts of the world tell me that they realized that it was important to deal with their trauma issue but they could not afford it, and living had to come first.

An additional structural reinforcement parameter is time. Some people are just so busy balancing a full-time (or two part-time) jobs, spouse, kids, aging parents that have needs, and similar very concrete concerns, that committing to psychotherapy is a challenge. The direct positive and negative reinforcement effects of these very concrete concerns overwhelm what psychotherapy can usually offer. For example, the emotional benefits of having a solid job and maintaining a marriage as positive reinforcement, and reduced adversity by preventing the stress of unemployment and divorce or isolation, negative reinforcement. One strategy that I have used in this regard is working one evening per week, to make it much easier for clients for whom busy work schedules preclude daytime visits. Several clients have reported that this helped a great deal and made it feasible to attend and progress. Another strategy is to promote the benefits of psychotherapy, although selling it is not ideal and there can be a thin line. One subtle approach is to indicate that resolution or improvement of mental health issues almost always improves functioning in more concrete areas of life, such as enhanced career and relationship success, and so is worth the time. Another approach is to use the "airplane oxygen" analogy: when the oxygen mask drops placing it on yourself first helps the survival of your kids. Likewise, taking care of your mental health assists those in your life.

Other structural components can play a role in reinforcement parameters, and some favor psychotherapy. For instance, a client's employer, spouse, or friend encouraging the individual to seek psychotherapy, issues related to this also addressed in the Motivation chapter. Both positive and negative reinforcement apply, depending on the given scenario. For example, improved feedback from the employer following mental health gains derived from psychotherapy (positive reinforcement), and being taken off work probation linked to impaired performance (negative reinforcement). Likewise, maintaining a romance or friendship with the emotional support and elimination or reduction of loneliness.

Regardless of the source of the structural variant of reinforcement parameters, both the therapist and client can play a role in the outcome.

Therapist Role

First and foremost, appreciate the importance and potency of reinforcement parameters! They are easy to miss or under value, and unless your training involves behavioral therapy techniques, you are unlikely to be thinking along this line. If the reinforcement parameters can be modified to favor psychotherapy, then take the steps to do so. For example, be flexible and adjust your schedule to accommodate clients, within reason. As a humorous anecdote, I heard of a therapist who apparently, or hopefully, was a "night owl" accommodating clients suffering from insomnia with 2:00 AM to 5:00 AM sessions! Another strategy is to promote, without overt selling, psychotherapy by pointing out the benefits that are often not as salient as concrete concerns in the lives of clients. The airplane oxygen analogy can help. Ultimately, though, if the structural reinforcement parameters do not favor psychotherapy, do not push for it. In the instance of my five clients not progressing to jobs and self-improvement despite being young, if I had my current experience and knowledge, I would have suggested that psychotherapy is not for them, at least now, and only follow the few on medication for prescription renewals. Of course, the Premier of Ontario unknowingly solved the failure to progress in psychotherapy problem for me!

It has been noted that the therapist can be an important source of social reinforcement for clients, derived from various factors such as personality, role behavior, value system, and skills (Krasner, 1962). Regarding personality, being open to experience as a therapist will strengthen a client's willingness to experiment with change. Adhering to behavior consistent with the professional role of therapist provides clients with confidence in addressing their issues and progressing. The therapist's value system can reinforce that of the client's when they align, such as expressing social justice concerns that the client resonates with. Skills enable the therapist to adjust the approach to what works for a given client, thereby advancing their wellbeing.

Client Role

As with therapists, appreciate and identify the structural reinforcement parameters acting in your life. In some instances, these can be adjusted to favor psychotherapy. For example, I have had clients say that they attended sessions with a psychologist or other type of psychotherapist, but when the insurance ran out they took the time and made the effort to seek out a psychiatrist covered by the government plan who does psychotherapy, and not just medication. In systems where no psychotherapy or limited is covered, some psychotherapists use sliding scales of client's income to payments, enhancing the affordability. If psychotherapy becomes cost effective then the structural reinforcement parameters related to financing shift in favor of it. Of tremendous importance, place value on your mental health and do not sacrifice it to the actual or perceived demands of existence. Regarding the former, apply the airplane oxygen analogy given that improvements to your mental health will have ripple effects in other areas, and for perceived demands realize that we live in a hyper-consumption society and can all get by with much less, the savings being applied to psychotherapy.

PSYCHOPATHOLOGY

Various forms of psychopathology can involve reinforcement parameters impacting on progress in psychotherapy, and in particular emotion-based disorders (depression, anxiety, and anger related), and addictions.

Emotion-Based Disorders

In the Motivation chapter, I presented the Amplification Effect: the evolution of human intelligence has made the cognitive activating appraisals underlying emotions more intensive, extensive, and added a temporal dimension, thereby amplifying emotions. This amplification process contributes to sadness transforming into depression, fear into anxiety, and anger into aggression problems (Bowins, 2004). Another key aspect of this amplification is mutually reinforcing (strengthening) negative cycles of thoughts and emotions, mentioned at the start of this chapter. In the case of sadness and depression, loss-related thoughts intensify feelings of sadness, which in turn create an emotional climate conducive to further loss related thoughts, leading to more sadness, and so on and so forth. With fear and anxiety, threat and danger cognitions strengthen feelings of fear, creating a feeling state favoring perceptions of threat and danger, and hence more fear, ensuring that specific fears amplify to anxiety. In the case of anger, perceptions of violation or damage increase feelings of anger, generating an emotional climate conducive to further perceptions of violation or damage, then intensified feelings of anger (Bowins, 2004). Therapists often describe these mutually reinforcing interactions between thoughts and emotions as negative feedback cycles, but reinforcement with strengthening of both components is really what is happening.

The key in psychotherapy is to neutralize this mutual reinforcement between negative thoughts and emotions, and then shift it from negative to positive. This process involves the concept of regulation and what I have referred to as "cognitive regulatory control therapies" (Bowins, 2013). The notion being that healthy psychological regulation, over in this instance thoughts and emotions, is impaired leading to the out of control amplification. The feel of this from a therapist's perspective, is that the client is almost locked into negativity with these mutually reinforcing feedback loops. Conceptualizing therapy as helping the client reestablish healthy regulation targets the interventions. To achieve this a combination of two strategies is optimal, the first being to pull the client away from this cycle via absorption in positive foci. Absorption is a mild beneficial form of dissociation (see the Impaired States and Processes for Mental Health chapter), and simply consists of immersion in positivity (Bowins, 2004, 2006). The range of options is unlimited, such as absorption in a good book, an interesting online video, exercise, a hobby, and even research. Various forms of meditation likely work in this fashion (Bowins, 2004). Absorption in positivity in a sense short-circuits the mutually reinforcing cycle of negative thoughts and emotions.

The second strategy, although both need to be addressed together, is reframing negative thoughts to positive ones. The focus is on shifting this negative spin into a positive direction, which entails an understanding that there is always a spin as advertisers know well, and with depression, anxiety, and anger problems, the spin is negative. Mental health can be conceptualized not as the absence of cognitive bias, but the presence of a skewed positivity bias (Beck, 1991; Beck & Clark, 1997). Beck (1991) states that the greatest explanatory power is provided by a model stipulating that (a) the non-depressed cognitive organization has a positive bias, (b) as it shifts toward depression, the cognitive bias is neutralized, (c) as depression develops, a negative bias occurs. It is help-ful to have clients become aware of their negative thoughts pertaining to loss, threats/danger, and violations/damage, and write them down. Then start prac-ticing negative to positive reframing, with the assistance of the therapist. For example, the thought "Everything in my life sucks," involves losses and pro-duces feelings of sadness and even despair. Having the client examine aspects of their life that function well is important. For instance, "My physical health is good," "I have a caring partner," I am retaining my job." Unlike with actual cognitive therapy, formal assignments are not required, and I have found that clients can work on this right in sessions without writing anything down. The more positive thoughts a person can generate the more the likely it is that the mutually reinforcing cycle between negative thoughts and emotions will shift to a positive cycle.

From the perspective of progress in psychotherapy, mutually reinforcing negative feedback loops create major impediments, ensuring that the client is immersed and even stuck in negativity. Neutralizing this process and shifting to mutually reinforcing cycles of positive thoughts and emotions can mas-sively advance progress in psychotherapy. An example pertaining to anger and aggression will illustrate this process. A late 30s client, Gino, presented with anger issues, psychotherapy motivated by his girlfriend, and also a sense that he was stuck in a negative angry mode. He clearly perceived the world in terms of violations and potential attacks, generating anger, ensuring further percep-tions of violation, and so on and so forth. The origins of his outlook and anger were not difficult to ascertain, Gino's father the key source. His father grew up in a difficult time period in another country without any positive support, and was very aggressive. The aggression included hitting Gino and his siblings for infractions, taking some swipes at his wife, and deliberately running over dogs on roads while Gino sat in the front seat of the truck. Gino ended up in many fights during school and weight lifted to become a stronger fighter. Unable to function in a "civilized" workplace, he entered into a rough business where the most optimal response to coworkers often started with "F you ..." and the like.

The starting point was immersion in positive pursuits like reading and music, which helped remove him from the negative mutually reinforcing thought-emotion cycles. At the same time, we began identifying the nature of his emotional information processing distortion, perceptions of violation and potential attacks triggering feelings of anger. He was able to see this quite clearly, and how thoughts and feelings strengthened one another. Although it took a short while, consistent with non-linear progress in therapy (see the Expectations chapter), he really took to the approach of identifying violation themed thoughts and reframing them to not see violations. These changes were evidenced by a much calmer, less rough, and more thoughtful demeanor. One day he stated that he had to quit his job as he could no longer stand the anger and aggression, and shortly shifted into a more benign job setting that enabled him to advance. Therapy progressed to dealing with the abuse issues, and the very accurate perception of violation over the treatment by his father, that of course fueled the anger. The transformation from an angry aggressive man to calm and thoughtful person was quite remarkable, and would never have occurred if he remained stuck in the mutually reinforcing cycle of violation themed thoughts and angry feelings.

Even though the discussion of emotion-based disorders has covered interventions, a brief note regarding the role of the therapist and client is warranted.

Therapist Role

Whenever emotional issues such as sadness-depression, fear-anxiety, and anger-aggression, are involved, recognize the emotional information processing aspect, amplification of negative emotions into disorders, and the role of mutually reinforcing cycles of negative thoughts and emotions in further amplifying the problem. Even if not familiar with cognitive techniques and assignments, appreciate that this approach can be informal without homework assignments, and apply the techniques described above. It is helpful to conceptualize the problem as impaired psychological regulation over emotional information processing, and think of restoring that regulation via, first, absorption in positivity to short circuit the negative cycles, and second, reframing the underlying thoughts. Also, realize that progress can and often is non-linear with a learning curve and limited progress followed by rapid advances. Some therapists in considering the example of Gino will comment that the abuse issues needed to be focused on at the start, but this can be a mistake as such issues are so emotionally charged that when Gino was immersed in the violation perception-anger/ aggression mode, too much anger might have arisen and ironically worsened the problem. He was more capable of dealing with this emotionally charged component of his problem when he had a solid handle on anger and aggression. The same concern can apply to sadness-depression and fear-anxiety problems.

Client Role

Intense negative feelings and being locked into mutually reinforcing cycles of negative thoughts and emotions, can and often do leave a person feeling powerless to do anything about it, being swept along by the negative current. Appreciate that by understanding emotional information processing and working with it, powerlessness can and usually does shift to empowerment. An advantage of emotional information processing conceptualizations is that they are very straightforward and logical, in contrast to the seemingly incoherent nature of emotions: loss—sadness, threat and danger—fear, violations and damage—anger. What could be more straightforward with the advantage of being completely accurate? Adding an understanding of the amplification of these emotions to depression, anxiety, and aggression via excessive negative thoughts, and the mutual reinforcement (strengthening) between these thoughts and feelings, transforms muddiness into clarity, and provides a clear path to improvement. Viewing emotions in this fashion and reframing negative perspectives to positive ones, preferably applying this strategy between sessions for real solid gains, can be very effective. Also, do not discount the power of absorption in positive activities, because although simple it pulls a person away from negativity helping to interrupt the mutually reinforcing cycles between negative thoughts and feelings. Of interest, I have found that some people struggle with cognitive reframing, even informal versions not requiring actual homework assignments, but have yet to encounter a client who cannot absorb themselves in a positive focus.

Addictions

Addiction problems impair functioning resulting in many setbacks in life, and clients need to advance with these issues if their functionality and success are to improve. Addiction problems also hinder progress with other mental illness concerns, such as depression, anxiety, abuse/trauma, and to advance with the latter necessitates success with the former. Tied into so-called addiction issues are a slew of related psychological problems, including self-concept and self-esteem, such that failure to progress with "addiction" problems greatly impedes overall progress in psychotherapy. The reason why I mention so-called addiction issues, and place addiction in quotations, is that the real issue is reinforcement (Bowins, 2016).

The terms addiction, impulse control, and compulsion (not linked to obsessions) are applied to the same behaviors adding confusion. Distinctions between these terms are arbitrary and do not hold out on close examination (see the Reinforcement-Based Disorders chapter of my book *Mental Illness Defined: Continuums, Regulation, and Defense* for a comprehensive coverage of this topic). Confusing overlap is evidenced in the descriptions applied to addictions, impulse control, and compulsions. For example, impulsivity consisting of unplanned responding and hasty decisions is a key shared marker of addictions (Clark, 2014). Impaired response inhibition plays a major role in compulsive enactments and also makes it difficult to prevent "addictive" responses (Clark, 2014; Grant et al., 2010). Diagnostic systems struggle to classify disorders as addictions, impulse control problems, or compulsions (American Psychiatric Association, 2013; First et al., 2002; World Health Organization, 1992). Reframing such problems as reinforcement-based not only captures the essence of what is transpiring, and hence, is more scientific, but greatly simplifies the understanding. Additionally, "addiction" problems have extended to computer-based entities, with changes in technology and the precise behavioral problem pertaining to it proceeding much faster than diagnostic systems can keep up with (Bowins, 2016). In the "good old days" with only alcohol, cocaine and the like, new "addiction" problems were almost unheard of, and if they emerged such as with stimulant medication abuses, there was time to research and classify them, but no longer with the pace of technological change, and even designer drugs. Hence, having a flexible format for describing and work-ing therapeutically with these reinforcement-based problem is greatly needed.

My solution to this need is a model including reinforcement, frequency of the behavior, intensity, and cost/benefits (Bowins, 2016). Regarding reinforcement, every instance of addictive, impulsive, and compulsive behavior involves pos-itive and/or negative reinforcement. For instance, excessive alcohol consump-tion feels good during the initial stimulant phase (positive reinforcement), and can relieve adverse emotional states (negative reinforcement). Likewise, sexual "addictions" are gratifying during the enactment, and often relieve feelings of boredom, emptiness, and loneliness, at least temporarily. The proposed model suggests rating positive and negative reinforcement on separate scales, with 1 the lowest amount and 10 the highest (or 1–5, 1–7, etc. as long as the same range is applied to each parameter). It is very important to separate positive and negative reinforcement because they are distinct and can lead to different interventions. For example, if positive reinforcement is high for a problematic behavior finding rewarding substitutes can help. If negative reinforcement is pronounced, address the underlying negative state relieved by the behavior, such as anxiety or loneliness, and then resolve it.

Frequency of the behavior is important, as if infrequent it is much less of a problem than if repeated regularly. For instance, occasional cocaine usage might not be much of a concern, whereas everyday use will be. A few drinks of alcohol per day is far less of a concern than drinking at breakfast right through to bedtime. Frequency of the behavior can be rated on the 1–10 scale with 1 very infrequent and 10 high. Intensity of the behavior is somewhat more complicated as it entails the sub-dimensions of tolerance, withdrawal effects, cravings, conscious focus and attention to the substance or behavior, resistance to alteration as evidenced by the extent of rationalizing cognitive distortions, and capacity to inhibit the behavior (Bowins, 2016). For example, with Internet gambling the person can become accustomed to a certain level or dollar amount (tolerance) leading to escalation, experience withdrawal effects like feeling downcast when not engaging, crave the behavior if not partaking in it, be consumed by thoughts of it even to the point of interfering with daily activities, strongly resist changing the behavior by extensive rationalizations, and be unable to refrain from going online and gambling. I suggest ratings for each component and then average them for an overall intensity raring. Cost/benefits is interesting and important, because although clinicians often assume that there is no real advantage to "addictive" behavior, as positive and negative reinforcement suggest, there is often pluses and minuses. When benefits exceed costs, then the behavior is unlikely to be that problematic. An example of a benefit is tension reduction which is a common to substance and behavioral addictions. I suggest that all the costs and benefits be listed separately, and a ratio created, perhaps from 1 to 10 to maintain consistency, with 10 costs ≫ benefits, and 1 benefits ≫ costs. Since 10 on the other ratings is the worst scenario, setting it up as cost/benefits is optimal.

Of profound significance, this model firstly can be applied to any instance of possible behavioral excess and, secondly, offers strategies to remedy the problem. Regarding the former, a person might engage in what appears to be excessive use of social media of a certain form. By the time formal diagnostic systems can establish a discrete diagnosis and set criteria, this form of "addiction" no longer exists, but with the reinforcement-based model proposed it can be characterized immediately. If reinforcement effects both positive and negative are very strong, and coupled with excessive frequency interfering with healthier activities, high intensity, and costs substantially exceed benefits, then alterations are required. Ratings on the specific dimensions inform regarding the direction of interventions (Bowins, 2016). For example, if positive reinforcement is too intense find substitute rewarding behaviors, such as learning or relearning how to play a musical instrument, and with negative reinforcement resolve the underlying negative state, as with anxiety, depression, or boredom. If a problem is excessive frequency, then moderating the behavior might well suffice, and is often more acceptable to the client. Withdrawal effects can be managed by a gradual reduction in the behavior, mutually agreed upon between the client and therapist, or by applying exposure and response prevention with refrain from engaging enhancing control over the behavior. Cravings and being consumed by thoughts of the behavior can benefit from absorption in positive activities, that draw a person's mental focus away from the problematic behavior. Extension rationalizations (very common) ensuring resistance to change, such as moderation, can be targeted by cognitive approaches aimed at correcting the distortions that maintain the behavior.

Therapist Role

Question the discrete diagnostic system that prevails (American Psychiatric Association, 2013; First et al., 2002; World Health Organization, 1992, 2022). One of the key frustrations I experience is knowing that nature is organized continuously, and learning from theoretical research (and some empirical research) that mental health and illness variables are organized continuously, but seeing diagnostic systems perpetuated the fiction of discrete conditions. I am uplifted that more objective and biologically focused research supports a dimensional model of mental illness (Hudziak et al., 2014), but find it sad that the discrete model persists, first because it aligns with our desire to simplify information processes instead of accurately describing the entity, and second, in some instances supports pharmaceutical company marketing objectives (Bowins, 2014). Standing in contrast to these psychological and monetary biases is the logic behind natural occurrences being organized continuously, based on trait variation so crucial to natural selection: a range of traits is required for environmental circumstances to favor some and not others, providing natural selection advantages (Bowins, 2016). For example, if there were only discrete traits, such as extremely long or short beaks, natural selection cannot act; instead a range is required for the environment to favor a bird with just the right size beak for the flowers in a given environment, as with Darwin's Galapagos finches (Darwin, 1858). Random genetic mutation produces a range of expressions for a given trait that natural selection acts upon, favoring those most optimal for the particular environment. Hence, natural entities are organized in continuous fashion!

Shifting to what I believe is a far more accurate dimensional perspective on mental illness, will free you from the absurd and confusing emphasis on addiction, impulse control, and compulsion classifications, and numerous discrete conditions flowing from this focus. Adopting the reinforcement-based model proposed makes it fast and relatively simple to characterize any such problem, and affords ways to intervene based on the ratings. In this era of false truths, alternative realities, and the like let us at least keep science free of these biases!

Client Role

With the help of the therapist rate the behavior in question on the dimensions provided above. Intensity subdimensions of tolerance, withdrawal effects, cravings, conscious focus and attention to the substance or behavior, resistance to alteration as evidenced by the extent of rationalizing cognitive distortions, and capacity to inhibit the behavior, will almost certainly require some assistance. From the spectrum of ratings work with the therapist to target the problematic issues. Realize that with any reinforcement-based concern relapses are the norm, and the key is to learn from these setbacks instead of beat yourself up about them, applying this knowledge to ongoing efforts. Depending on the problem, and more specifically the social context, appreciate that people affiliate largely based on their substance and behavioral use/abuse patterns. For example, social drinkers tend to engage with lighter drinkers, hard core drinkers as "bar flies," and the like. I have subspecialty training and much experience with "addictions," and have found that this pattern holds remarkably well. Now when you alter your pattern, do not expect your "buddies" to change as it almost never occurs. Consequently, a major problem for a person trying to go "clean and sober" is isolation, often inducing negative emotions increasing the risk of relapse. This is why it is crucial to plug into a non (or similarly) using social network, such as Alcoholics Anonymous, Smart Recovery, or even emerging social media groups. The supportive social contact from nonusers goes a long way in progress with addiction therapy, and from this addressing underlying issues. I usually tell clients with these issues, "Managing the addiction itself is often the easy part, addressing the underlying issues more of a challenge, but the first leads to success with the latter." In line with this I have had many clients successfully progress with their mood, abuse/trauma, and other issues upon stabilizing and improving the reinforcement-based problem.

CODEPENDENCE

When two people, or potentially more, are completely dependent on one another, such that it is difficult to function independently or even imagine this, codependency exists. This scenario is quite common in the "addiction," or what I refer to as the reinforcement-based area, but can arise in any scenario. Reinforcement applies because both parties reinforce dependence in the other, hence the codependence. I will present a couple of case examples to illustrate how diverse the manifestations are.

Bill was in his mid-40s when he first attended showing significant anxiety and depression. He worked as a management consultant but was let go from the company a couple of years prior. He was clearly fearful of applying for jobs and avoidant. He indicated that he no longer liked the type of work, but this was a rationalization to a great extent, as given his experience he could have applied for related positions in the business world. His physical profile stood out because he was very overweight, with most of the excess in his mid-section. To manage the anxiety and depression an antidepressant was started, and we worked on the fear and avoidance issues but with very limited progress. After a substantial number of sessions, he opened up about his romance with another man. His partner was younger, athletic, more attractive, and quite demanding of Bill's attention. He revealed that his partner had a strong preference for overweight, even morbidly obese, somewhat older men. Apparently, there are organized meetups in the United States and elsewhere, where these overweight men get together and have sex with their admirers, events that Bill's partner had attended. One problem his virile partner faced was that many of these men could not function well sexually, but Bill definitely could. This greatly endeared Bill to his partner, and given the strength of his partner's interests in this regard, he became sexually dependent on Bill. Being insecure about his career and appearance, Bill became reliant on his younger and more attractive partner. This mutual dependency escalated, with Bill gaining weight to be more attractive to his partner, and wanting to be around him much of the time, in case his partner strayed. With the very pronounced weight Bill would not have presented well at any interview, which intensified the fear of applying for regular work. Bill wanted to lose weight to improve his health but said he could not risk his partner losing interest. His partner also relied on Bill for money saved through the years, but seemed ambivalent about Bill working, in a sense wanting him to work for money while also needing Bill's attention much of the time. The codependency was so great that nothing changed Bill's avoidance of work. Eventually, the relationship imploded when Bill's partner spent so much money that they had to sell their condo to break even, followed by his partner shifting to another overweight man he met. Bill left therapy at this point instead of trying to progress independently.

A much different codependent scenario occurred with Jasmine, a mid-20s woman with anorexia. My experience with anorexia has not been positive and I am very reluctant to take such a client on, and never will unless they (almost always female) attend group therapy for eating disorders concurrently. A major problem with this condition is that there is a great deal of self and other deception pertaining to eating behavior, that is very difficult to overcome, in part because the person gains a sense of control from calorie counting and restricting, excessive exercise, laxative use, and the like, and deceives to maintain the behavior. Jasmine listened to my description of self and other deception, and agreed that she had acted like this but wanted change. Codependency occurred between herself and her parents, who insisted that she be at home when not at work, and she worked with her father. They seemed to be very fearful of her and also her sister moving on, and routinely commented on how Jasmine needs them and cannot cope on her own, pointing out how threatening the world is. She felt very insecure and relied on them for most things including work with her father. However, she had fantasies of a boyfriend, a family, travel, and more friends, prompting her to seek both group therapy and a psychiatrist. Early in her therapy nothing really happened with ongoing deceptions pertaining to her eating behavior, such as "I've let myself eat more" compensated equally by increasing exercise. No real progress occurred with the codependency either, Jasmine resisting the notion of significantly altering it. Seeing the same lack of progress, I suggested that we end sessions and she seek a therapist who specializes in eating disorders. This input apparently jolted her and she really engaged with therapy, talking about how she resented her parents treating her like a child and blocking her maturity. We went over how she had to take charge and empower herself, instead of just exert control over eating behavior. She allowed herself to gain weight and for the first time had menstrual periods. She started dating, decided to look for another job not with a family member, and worked on plans to travel. The change was very pleasing to see, along with reports of her feeling better. Then it all fell apart! Her parents launched a major campaign to reinforce her insecurities and convince her that all these steps will lead to disaster. I suggested family counseling, something proposed at the start but rejected. She missed a couple of sessions and refused to pay for even one, indicating how uncaring I am as a therapist. Inadvertently a year later I received a report from her eating disorder program, confirming that ever gain made was lost.

These two case examples, and I have more like them, have convinced me that trying to take on intensely codependent clients is usually not worth the output of time and effort, although successful outcomes can transpire with mild to moderate codependency. My approach now is to present the interpretation to the codependent client and gauge the reaction. If the client seems less than highly motivated to deal with the codependency problem, I suggest couple or family therapy.

Therapist Role

Be vigilant for codependent scenarios and realize that if one exists then there is a major barrier to psychotherapy progress. Appreciate that codependency can take many forms, and also that it can take time to reveal itself in therapy.

From my experience and that of other therapists spoken with, the effort is usually not worth the abysmal gain, at least when the problem is to the intense end of the spectrum. I believe that it is best to address the codependency with the client and only progress, or progress further, if the person seems really committed, but therapy can still falter as with Jasmine. It is best to suggest couple or family therapy, as when the codependent parties are present in sessions progress is more likely. Interestingly, the only codependent scenarios where I have made significant inroads are with "addiction" clients who have quite a bit of clean and sober time. They realize from AA meetings (and other 12-Step programs) that codependence is common with these problems, the "addict" relying on an insecure person who enables their alcohol/drug usage to keep them needy. Being aware of this problem they seem more open to changing the scenario, which in a major sense is already changed by no longer using the substance.

Client Role

Be open to the interpretation that codependency is occurring and do not rationalize it. If not committed to changing the paradigm, then psychotherapy is unlikely to work out well. The best option even if more committed is couple or family therapy, depending on who the codependent person or people are, because issues with both parties that reinforce the mutual dependency can be addressed in this context. As mentioned under the therapist role, substance abuse issues seem to offer more hope so long as the person has significant clean and sober time.

SUMMARY NOTE

Reinforcement parameters are very interesting in that they potently impact on psychotherapy progress, while often hidden and/or ignored. Structural parameters such as money and time can be deal breakers for therapy, and are worth making the effort to manage, with flexibility such as sliding payment scales and accommodating the client's schedule within reason paramount. Regarding psychopathology, mutually reinforcing cycles of negative thoughts and emotions keep clients locked into sadness-depression, fear-anxiety, and anger-aggression problems. Neutralizing them through absorption in positive foci, and cognitive reframing to facilitate a shift from negative to positive mutual reinforcement, is crucial for psychotherapy progress with these common problems. "Addictions" constitute a major form of reinforcement parameter, and reframing them as reinforcement-based disorders provides a more accurate characterization. Applying the proposed rating system emphasizing positive and negative reinforcement, frequency of the behavior, intensity of the behavior, and costs/benefits, assists in rapidly characterizing a wide range of these problems, and provides strategies for targeting the main problem areas. Codependency presents a major barrier to psychotherapy progress due to the mutual and often escalating reinforcement. Couple or family therapy is the best option, aside from some "addiction" scenarios. Reinforcement, much like the seas for sailors, can powerfully work for or against therapy, and addressing potent adverse scenarios will advance psychotherapy progress.

REFERENCES

American Psychiatric Association. (2013). *Diagnostic & statistical manual 5*. American Psychiatric Publishing Inc.

Beck, A. (1991). Cognitive therapy: A 30-year retrospective. *American Psychologist, 46*(4), 368–375.

Beck, A., & Clark, D. (1997). An information processing model of anxiety: Automatic and strategic processes. *Behavior Research and Therapy, 35*(1), 49–58.

Bowins, B. E. (2004). Psychological defense mechanisms: A new perspective. *American Journal of Psychoanalysis, 64*, 1–26.

Bowins, B. E. (2006). How psychiatric treatments can enhance psychological defense mechanisms. *American Journal of Psychoanalysis, 66*, 173–194.

Bowins, B. E. (2013). Cognitive regulatory control therapies. *American Journal of Psychotherapy, 67*(3), 215–236.

Bowins, B. E. (2014). *At the tipping point: How to save us from self-destruction*. Infinity.

Bowins, B. E. (2016). *Mental illness defined: Continuums, regulation, and defense*. Routledge.

Clark, L. (2014). Disordered gambling: The evolving concept of behavioral addiction. *Annals of The New York Academy of Science, 1327*, 46–61.

Darwin, C. (1858). *On the origin of species*. Signet Classics.

First, M. B., Frances, A., & Pincus, H. A. (2002). *DSM-IV-TR handbook of differential diagnosis*. American Psychiatric Publishing Inc.

Grant, J. E., Potenza, M. N., Weinstein, A., & Gorelick, D. A. (2010). Introduction to behavioral addictions. *American Journal of Drug & Alcohol Abuse, 36*(5), 233–241.

Hudziak, J. J., Albaugh, M. D., Ducharme, S., Karama, S., Spottswood, M., Crehan, E., et al. (2014). Cortical thickening maturation and duration of music training: Health-promoting activities shape brain development. *Journal of the American Academy of Child and Adolescent Psychiatry, 53*(11), 1153–1161.

Krasner, L. (1962). The therapist as a social reinforcement machine. In H. H. Strupp & L. Luborsky (Eds.), *Research in psychotherapy* (pp. 61–94). American Psychological Association.

World Health Organization. (1992). *The ICD-10 classification of mental and behavioral disorders: Clinical descriptions and diagnostic guidelines*. World Health Organization.

World Health Organization. (2022). *The ICD-10 classification of mental and behavioral disorders: Clinical descriptions and diagnostic guidelines*. World Health Organization.

Chapter 5

COMPLEXITY

It is usually the case that the more complex a problem is the harder it is to solve, and at least at face value this would appear to be the case for psychotherapy. In the Personality Disorders chapter, we looked at how severe expressions of these conditions can be very challenging and the severity is an impediment to progress. An extreme expression of Avoidant Personality Disorder often results in the client avoiding psychotherapy when faced with any stressful or challenging issue. Narcissistic Personality Disorder is in my experience one of the most difficult conditions to treat, particularly when intense, because the vulnerability side leaves the client so sensitive that it can feel like navigating a minefield for the therapist, and the compensatory side so excessive that it is difficult to contend with. In the instance of Dependent Personality Disorder, severe dependence as is seen in many codependent scenarios, greatly reduces the probability of real progress to independence. Clients with Obsessive-Compulsive Personality Disorder can be so rutted in their compulsive behavior that significant change is difficult to achieve. Antisocial Personality Disorder is largely resilient to modification, given the evolution as a deceit-based strategy utilizing dissociation, such that the person often deceives themselves about their deception capacity. Severe Borderline Personality Disorder makes progress with one-to-one therapy very unlikely, and this intensity usually requires an initial group intervention to help the client regulate emotions and self-harm behavior to the point that individual psychotherapy can be tolerated (Links et al., 2017). Compounding the problem is a high level of reactivity (neuroticism) that amplifies the impact of trauma, and intensifies Borderline Personality Disorder symptoms. High reactivity also intensifies most other mental illness conditions, making them less amendable to psychotherapy. Hence, in the case of personality disorders greater complexity derived from more severe manifestations does impede progress in psychotherapy.

For mental illness manifestations other than personality disorders, increasing complexity can impede psychotherapy progress. We will now look at how this plays out for comorbidity, severity, and practical psychotherapy issues such as attendance and scheduling.

DOI: 10.4324/b23346-6

COMORBIDITY

When mental illness occurs in combinations there is greater complexity, but does this impede progress in psychotherapy? In contrast to more severe expressions of personality disorders where there is an intuitive logic and the experience of most psychotherapists, combinations of conditions is not so intuitive. Let us see what the literature indicates. We will look at revealing studies finding that comorbidity is an impediment and research finding that it is not.

Research Finding That Comorbidity Impedes Psychotherapy Progress

Some research supports the notion that comorbidity does impede progress with psychotherapy. Brown et al. (1996) examined 157 primary care patients who met criteria for major depression, randomly assigning them to interpersonal psychotherapy or antidepressant treatment. At baseline and four and eight months they assessed for severity of depression and anxiety disorders. Patients with comorbid depression and anxiety presented with significantly more psychopathology and were more likely to terminate treatment prematurely. However, psychotherapy and antidepressant treatments were effective for the depressed patients with and without comorbidity, although time to recovery was longer in the comorbid group (Brown et al., 1996). Reviewing the literature, Lecrubier (1998) focused on panic disorder comorbidity. Panic disorder on its own was not common compared to other mental illnesses, such as depression. Comorbidity of panic disorder (attacks) resulted in more severe anxiety and depressive symptoms, a higher rate of suicide attempts, and poorer response and compliance to various treatments including psychotherapy.

Panic attacks as a more severe scenario ties into the all-important topic of the discrete or continuous nature of psychopathology, and from this understanding what comorbidity actually consists of. As mentioned previously, anxiety and depression are continuous in nature, in contrast to the portrayal in major diagnostic systems (American Psychiatric Association, 2013; First et al., 2002; World Health Organization, 1992, 2022). Based on my research, they range in terms of severity and duration, with the most severe manifestations yielding seemingly distinct manifestations as an emergent property; quantitative variation providing the impression of qualitative variation (Bowins, 2015, 2016). In the case of depression, "melancholic depression" occurs with vegetative features, but this is only a severe expression of depression. A hundred years of depression research has not produced a distinct type that has held up to scrutiny (Bowins, 2015), strongly suggesting that we relinquish this pursuit, but yet each new installment of the major diagnostic editions comes out with different discrete types (American Psychiatric Association, 2013; First et al., 2002; World Health Organization, 1992, 2022). Postulated types of depression only constitute eliciting circumstances that can somewhat shape the presentation, such as hypothyroidism contributing to fatigue and motor slowness.

Anxiety is more difficult to conceptualize from a continuous perspective, but a starting point is that if depression based on the root emotion of sadness is continuous, it follows that anxiety based on another primary emotion—fear—will also be continuous. Furthermore, the emotional information processing core circumstances of sadness and fear overlap, as loss circumstances (sadness) often entail threat and danger (fear), and vice versa. For example, a person about to be terminated from a good job perceives a threat and loss, triggering fear and sadness. Indeed, due to these considerations it is almost inconceivable that depression is continuous and anxiety not. Anxiety, in my opinion, is continuous with the most extreme range yielding panic attacks as an emergent property, derived from activation of the fight/flight/freeze response (Bowins, 2016). A potential critique is that anxiety does seem to come in various forms, such as social, phobias, generalized, and panic. Panic is a more severe expression derived from the fight/flight/freeze response, and occurs in many conditions including other "forms" of anxiety and depression (Lecrubier, 1998). The other supposedly discrete forms really arise from eliciting circumstances, that can shape the presentation. For example, social scenarios elicit "social anxiety" and the circumstance shapes the expression, such as avoidance of social encounters, interpersonal sensitivity, and social status manifestations. Non-social threats such as heights and spiders trigger phobias, that influence the presentation as with avoiding heights and marked physiological responses to the triggering agent. Likewise, more cognitive threats produce "generalized" anxiety with worry. Each of these supposed forms of anxiety can vary in severity with the most severe expressions triggering panic attacks. A closer look reveals the absurdity of discrete types, as why a specific non-social threat constitutes a phobia, and a social threat social anxiety, and why is a "social phobia" somehow different than a regular phobia? Also, worry-based anxiety is generalized, assuming that there is more than one focus, but why is this different than several specific object and social sources of threat, with more foci producing a more severe expression? Of interest and relevance, worry is continuous in distribution, having an equal association with anxiety, stress, and depression, and so is not restricted to "generalized" anxiety (Olatunji et al., 2010a).

Anxiety represents the core, based on the root emotion of fear that relies on the same basic neural processing, although different areas of the brain are additionally activated with the given eliciting circumstances, such as social status and attachment processing with "social" anxiety (Bowins, 2016). Hence, clearing away the conceptual confusion demonstrates that depression and anxiety are continuous, with the most severe manifestations yielding seemingly distinct "types" as an emergent property, melancholic presentations in the case of depression, and panic attacks with anxiety. Varying expressions of depression and anxiety arise from eliciting circumstances that somewhat shape the presentation, although for each condition the core emotional information processing and related neural mechanisms are shared. Depression and anxiety continuums often interface due to the emotional information processing overlap, and the interfacing of continuums is what accounts for comorbidity. Supporting this overlap, Goldstein-Piekarski et al. (2016) found in a study of anxiety disorder comorbidity that 60% of those with an anxiety disorder had another anxiety disorder or depression. In addition to depression and anxiety continuums that interface producing comorbidity, others can as well such as hypomania-mania, psychosis, dissociation, reinforcement-based disorders (addictions), and eating disorders—for an extensive coverage of this topic and anxiety as a continuum see Bowins (2016). Interfacing of these continuums is integral to comorbidity.

Getting back to the research finding that comorbidity impedes psychotherapy progress, Siegfried (1998) conducted a review study of a very common comorbidity—substance abuse and major mental illness—finding that it is associated with poorer outcomes. Focusing on depression and personality disorder comorbidity, Shea et al. (1992) in a review study determined that the presence of personality disorders was associated with a poorer response to treatment. Reuter et al. (2016) also found that in their sample of 546 inpatients, a comorbid personality disorder constituted a consistent predictor of psychotherapy nonresponse. Examining childhood comorbidity involving anxiety, Walczak et al. (2018) identified and reviewed 33 publications based on 28 randomized controlled trials, and even though there was a mixture of results, they concluded that comorbidity has a more negative outcome than previous reviews suggest. The studies examined here indicate that there is some definite evidence supporting the position that comorbidity impedes psychotherapy (and other treatment) progression.

Research Finding That Comorbidity Does Not Impede Psychotherapy Progress

As is common in research where there is not an absolute answer, such as the mass of an object, there is a mixture of results with several psychotherapy studies finding that comorbidity does not have a significant impact on outcomes. Gersh et al. (2017) conducted a systematic review and meta-analysis of dropout rates in individual psychotherapy for generalize anxiety disorder, with 45 studies involving 2,224 participants. The mean dropout rate was 17% with quite a bit of variability, but comorbid conditions did not influence the outcome (Gersh et al., 2017). Another study of generalized anxiety disorder by Newman et al. (2010) involved 76 participants receiving cognitive and behavioral therapies, with other anxiety disorders and depression comorbidity evaluated. They found that comorbidity resulted in greater treatment response! Given that this is an isolated study, not a review of studies, it would have to be replicated, but is suggestive that comorbidity does not necessarily impede psychotherapy progress and might even yield better outcomes. Demonstrating that a mix of results is often the norm, Olatunji et al. (2010b) came up with results that varied with the diagnosis: their meta-analysis of 148 anxiety disorder treatment samples involving cognitive behavioral therapy, dynamic therapy, mindfulness, and biological treatments, revealed that while comorbidity associated with "neurotic" anxiety samples impaired treatment outcomes, comorbidity involving panic disorder and/or agoraphobia with Post-Traumatic Stress Disorder (PTSD) or sexual abuse did not impede progress. Regarding personality disorder comorbidity, Van Bronswijk et al. (2018) focusing on depression randomized 146 patients to either cognitive therapy or interpersonal psychotherapy, finding that the dropout rate was not impacted by personality disorder comorbidity. Note how this contrasts with the results of Shea et al. (1992) and Reuter et al. (2016) mentioned in the prior section.

The studies discussed so far have involved adult samples. Ollendick et al. (2008) conducted a review of youth anxiety, affective, Attention Deficit Hyperactivity Disorder (ADHD), and oppositional/conduct problem comorbidity. They found that comorbidity is the rule and not the exception, and that in general it does not negatively impact on treatment outcome, although there was variability in the studies examined. Clearly there is research support for both comorbidity not impeding psychotherapy progress and impeding it. There are no definitive studies and so no definitive answers, and it might come down to specific individuals or even samples, but a potential option is severity that we will look at after a mention of what therapists and clients can do regarding comorbidity.

Therapist Role

Based on the mix of results, do not assume that comorbidity necessarily contributes to a worse outcome, as the verdict is not in. Also, the mix of outcomes in even the same study suggests that several factors play a role in whether or not comorbidity impedes psychotherapy outcomes. To optimize outcomes, firstly, be optimistic that success can transpire. Second, do a thorough assessment to determine what conditions pertain to the given client. Third, be open to seeing that there is another condition not initially assessed, as quite commonly another will emerge during therapy. For example, after recovering or significantly improving from depression, Narcissistic Personality Disorder might become evident. Fourth, strategize treatment to manage each condition. Eclectic psychotherapy is of value with comorbidity, because clients with greater complexity due to comorbidity will often require diverse interventions.

Client Role

Be open to the possibility that more than one problem exists. People frequently rationalize occurrences in a self-enhancing fashion as part of the positive cognitive distortion form of psychological defense (Bowins, 2004, 2006). The most comfortable reason for a problem is often held onto and others rejected. I have noted this very frequently where personality disorders are concerned: "I have depression, my personality is fine." Responses of this nature indicate that the client is rationalizing their issues as something more socially acceptable than a personality disorder. Likewise, depression, anxiety, and substance abuse are commonly cited to rationalize psychotic symptoms, and often more by distressed parents than the client. Although it can be painful, clear away the rationalizations and listen to what the therapist is proposing. I have seen many clients with comorbid conditions improve in terms of depression or anxiety, but then reject the notion of another issue, only to walk away with persistent personality and/or substance abuse issues, invariably returning to me or another psychotherapist when depression or anxiety (or both) arise again, due largely to the comorbid condition. In some instances, these futile cycles repeat endlessly. By accepting that more than one problem is occurring and addressing each in therapy real enduring progress can transpire.

SEVERITY

Given how comorbidity per se does not necessarily block progress with psychotherapy, it might be severity that is paramount. We noted this for personality disorders (see the Personality Disorders chapter), and how based on a systemic review of 18 psychotherapy studies, outcomes are better with a higher level of personality organization, and worse with poorer personality organization (Koelen et al., 2012). Goddard et al. (2015) studied psychotherapy clients as part of the United Kingdom's Improving Access to Psychological Treatments initiative, to provide access to evidence based psychological interventions for mild to moderate mental health problems in a primary care setting. They applied a prospective cohort design with 1,249 participants. Higher scores for personality disorder linked to poorer outcomes in terms of depression, anxiety, and social functioning, and reduced recovery rates at the end of psychotherapy (Goddard et al., 2015). Focusing on cognitive-behavioral therapy for "health anxiety," Sanatinia et al. (2016) examined 381 patients, 86% having some personality dysfunction and 41% meeting the criteria for a personality disorder. More severe personality disorder manifestations resulted in less benefit from psychotherapy. Interestingly, the absence of any personality problem translated into a reduced response to the CBT intervention for the condition focused on, whereas those with less than severe personality problems showed greater improvements over two years (Sanatinia et al., 2016). Hence, as pertains to personality problems, greater severity does impede psychotherapy progress, whereas mild to moderate manifestations can progress well. This conclusion based on research aligns with my clinical experience, as I have had many clients with mild to moderate personality disorders (antisocial excluded) progress very well with psychotherapy, but severe expressions are a major impediment, at least until a group intervention improves their emotional and behavioral regulation.

Severity of depression and anxiety also seems relevant to progress with psychotherapy. Under Research Finding That Comorbidity Impedes

Psychotherapy Progress, we covered the review by Lecrubier (1998) focusing on panic disorder comorbidity, who found that comorbidity of panic disorder (the most severe expression of anxiety) results in more severe overall anxiety and depressive symptoms, higher rate of suicide attempts, and a poorer response and compliance to various treatments including psychotherapy. Premature termination from therapy (obviously impeding progress) for depression, anxiety, and other issues does seem to occur with higher severity of the given condition (Derisley & Reynolds, 2000). Severity need not relate directly to depression or anxiety but instead factors influencing psychotherapy. For example, Mohr et al. (1990) evaluated 62 patients receiving psychotherapy for major depression, finding that those who responded poorly were characterized by high levels of interpersonal difficulty that played into problems with psychotherapy.

As a psychiatrist using medication as well as psychotherapy, clients with severe depression and anxiety are often referred. Invariably, I have found that for such clients the combination of psychotherapy and medications (typically antidepressants and also benzodiazepines for panic attacks) works better than either alone. For milder manifestations, psychotherapy alone seems to be not only fine, but often superior. One of the key reasons for why the combination of psychotherapy and medications works so well, is that the severity of depression and anxiety can make it challenging for the client to engage with psychotherapy strategies such as cognitive reframing. Reduced depression and anxiety with medication treatment provides an elevated and solid base of emotional functioning, enabling the client to work with psychotherapy.

The only psychotherapy strategy that is really effective for severe depression is behavioral activation in a graded fashion, focusing on physical, social, and mental functioning. For instance, have the client simply get out of bed and sit on the couch to start. Listen to the radio or television for social input, and look at the front cover of a book for mental activity. Then the client progresses to more activity, such as walking in the house or apartment, responding to their partner, and maybe reading a child's book with big simple letters. As this example indicates, the challenge is much less intense than cognitive reframing, and unless a client is catatonic which is rarely seen, the person can advance with behavioral activation. Even then, a combination of this form of psychotherapy and medication is often optimal. Returning to the notion of non-linear change in psychotherapy (Hayes et al., 2007), it is important to realize that with more severe manifestations of mental illness change can be slower to come about, but will often proceed rapidly when the client's functioning stabilizes, particularly if this is accompanied by insight and motivation. Adversarial growth is a related consideration, transpiring when occurrences such as trauma act as a catalyst for extensive change (Hayes et al., 2007).

Severity does add complexity that can impede progress with psychotherapy, or treatment in general. Considering how impactful severity can be on psychotherapy progress what can the therapist and client do about it?

Therapist Role

Appreciate that complexity in terms of severe expressions of a given condition translates into worse psychotherapy outcomes, independent of your skill set. Therapists often tend to blame themselves for poor outcomes, based on what I have observed, and it is important to set the boundaries: if high severity typically means worse outcomes, this is what it is. Refrain from self-blame, and instead praise yourself if you succeed with a client who has a severe form of personality disorder, depression, anxiety, substance abuse, and really any condition. Do not try and be a hero or martyr as this is only good for one episode, and psychotherapy is your career. DO NOT burn yourself out. I have seen psychotherapists and social workers do this, only to exit the practice in a few years, which is sad as it can be avoided by setting the right parameters. As a brief client example, I was hoodwinked by another psychiatrist early in my practice, when she asked if I would take a client with Borderline Personality Disorder since she was moving out of Toronto. She expressed that the client is workable and has charming aspects. During the assessment, this client began punching the couch and shouting, demonstrating very poor regulation of emotions and aggression. I assertively expressed, "In my office displays of aggression are not allowed!" The tone perhaps more than the words stopped her cold, and she responded, "My prior therapist allowed this." You see how I was indeed hoodwinked! I replied, "Maybe that is so but not here, and I am going to end the assessment now. I advise that you go back to Dr. _____, and get a referral to a group therapy program for personality disorders." I had no intention of being a hero (or martyr) and setting the parameters was crucial. To confirm how severe her state was, not that any additional support is needed, she also expressed, "I've been angry ever since I was abused in the womb, which I clearly remember."

If your role as a psychotherapist does not include prescribing medication, and faced with severe depression and/or anxiety, it is best to seek out a psychiatrist who can prescribe. Appreciate that for severe expressions of these conditions, the combination of medication and psychotherapy usually works better than either alone! If faced with severe depression, anxiety, obsessive-compulsive, and other problems, and a client who is very resistant to medication, the best option is behavioral therapy strategies such as behavioral activation for depression, and exposure and response prevention for obsessive-compulsive issues.

Client Role

If you believe you have, or have been told that you have, a more severe form of a personality disorder, then ask yourself how committed you are to improvement. For those who are committed to improvement then some form of therapy is appropriate. If regulation over emotions and behavior such as aggression is an issue (very common in extreme personality disorders), then the starting point is group psychotherapy oriented to improving regulation. The one-to-one of individual psychotherapy is too much of a challenge, at least to start with. However, with improved regulation of emotions and behavior, individual psychotherapy is feasible as you now likely have a moderate level of the personality disorder. If the issue is severe depression and/or anxiety, be open to medication and possibly behavioral activation therapy. Also, do not discourage as I have had several clients with severe expressions of depression and/or anxiety progress very well in psychotherapy, at least when combined with medication.

PRACTICAL PSYCHOTHERAPY ISSUES

Features relevant to a given psychotherapy setting can add complexity that often translates into the client dropping out of therapy. These features can be diverse and unique, only sharing how they make it more difficult for the client to participate, thereby increasing dropout rates. For example, in my setting of Ontario, prior to the COVID-19 pandemic, regular telephone psychotherapy sessions were not allowed by the Ministry of Health. For most people living in the city core this was not much of a concern, but for clients attending from further out it became more of a problem with what might be called the "construction era" in Toronto. Condo buildings started to go up all over the city, with partial road blocks. Add in the rapidly expanding population, streets not designed to accommodate all the traffic, inadequate public transportation, and it became a real challenge for some clients to make it into sessions. One might wonder why they did not seek psychotherapy in their area? The answer often being that it was not available. Some were willing to face the long commute in and back, but others just dropped out. Calls for the government ministry to allow telephone sessions fell on deaf ears (other than for registering in a complex Internet system they control), with claims that this would not work well. However, with COVID-19 it was suddenly allowed and worked well. An interesting benefit of this pandemic then being that clients living further away could easily have a safe session. Ironically, given how empty the roads became, it would not have taken long at all for them to travel in even during "rush" hour. This example demonstrates how the way forward with more and more congested cities and pandemic scenarios, might well end up being "tele-psychotherapy." Based on my pandemic experience it works well, and one thing I noted during the pandemic was that almost no one missed a session or called in to cancel. Who knows, maybe some therapist or client reading this book in 50 years might exclaim, "Wow, they really had face to face sessions back then!"

Another variant of practical psychotherapy complexity pertains to the number of sessions required by the therapist. Some therapists require two sessions per week, and not just psychoanalysts, claiming that this is needed for progress. From my experience, even applying psychodynamic strategies, once per week is fine. While some clients can easily accommodate two and even more sessions per week, for many people more than once per week adds complexity that can increase the dropout rate. Homework assignments, such as occurs with cognitive behavioral therapy, comprise another source of complexity. Based on my experience, discussed earlier, many clients do not complete these assignments and feel bad for not doing so. An issue for CBT therapists is how to encourage and ensure that clients do the homework. Early in my practice I discovered that much less formal versions of cognitive and behavioral therapy (they are not always one and the same) reduces complexity, is much easier for clients for whom homework is not likely to be completed or even attempted, and the outcome seems fine. With this less formal approach, many clients stayed in therapy who would have dropped out if I insisted on the assignments being completed. I have had clients claim that they were "kicked out" of CBT for not doing the homework, although I did not substantiate the claims. What can therapists and clients do about these practical sources of psychotherapy complexity?

Therapist Role

The range of practical psychotherapy sources of complexity is such that you really have to examine your given practice to see what might apply. Ask clients how challenging it is for them to attend and partake, which ties into the benefit/cost ratio covered in the Motivation chapter. For some issues, such as my Toronto-based example of long distance commute times, there is really little that can be done, and it took a pandemic to change the options for clients. However, there are other sources of complexity that are possible to work with, such as the frequency and number of sessions, and any "homework" requirements. Exploring the option of "tele-psychotherapy" for clients who struggle to make it in might be the future of therapy.

Client Role

Try and be accommodating, particularly if the benefits of psychotherapy substantially exceed the costs. Prior to the pandemic, I often told long distance clients that Toronto has a lot to offer, and why not make it a morning or afternoon adding a visit to a restaurant, store, friend, or even walking around. Some followed this suggestion and the therapy half-day, or even full-day, became an interesting excursion. I also suggest that you listen to the therapist regarding what might be required, as there is often a reason based on experience, much like a mechanic recommending something for your car. If what is suggested adds too much complexity, then see if there is a compromise position. For example, I have negotiated with some clients for once every two-week therapy, which for intense issues such as trauma is not ideal but workable.

SUMMARY NOTE

Greater complexity in regard to client issues and practical aspects of psychotherapy, often translates into higher dropout rates and diminished likelihood of real progress. Comorbidity is seemingly a potent source of complexity, but as we have seen, research results are quite mixed regarding psychotherapy outcomes. Comorbid conditions are definitely not a deal breaker for psychotherapy, and by working on the applicable problems solid outcomes are viable. The real issue might not be comorbidity but severity. More severe manifestations of mental illness add complexity that can increase dropout rates and impede progress. Personality disorders are a clear example of how severity impacts on psychotherapy outcomes. Comorbidity and severity interact, in that if the comorbid conditions are severe, then psychotherapy progress is even less likely, whereas if the conditions fall in the mild to moderate range, more progress might occur than for one very severe condition. Practical psychotherapy issues can add complexity and can be relatively easy to manage, thereby reducing dropout rates.

REFERENCES

American Psychiatric Association. (2013). *Diagnostic & statistical manual 5*. American Psychiatric Publishing.

Bowins, B. E. (2004). Psychological defense mechanisms: A new perspective. *American Journal of Psychoanalysis, 64*, 1–26.

Bowins, B. E. (2006). How psychiatric treatments can enhance psychological defense mechanisms. *American Journal of Psychoanalysis, 66*, 173–194.

Bowins, B. E. (2015). Depression: Discrete or continuous? *Psychopathology, 48*(2), 69–78.

Bowins, B. E. (2016). *Mental illness defined: Continuums, regulation, and defense*. Routledge.

Brown, C., Schulberg, H. C., Madonia, M. J., Shear, M. K., & Houck, P. R. (1996). Treatment outcomes for primary care patients with major depression and lifetime anxiety disorders. *American Journal of Psychiatry, 153*(10), 1293–1300.

Derisley, J., & Reynolds, S. (2000). The transtheoretical stages of change as a predictor of premature termination, attendance and alliance in psychotherapy. *British Journal of Clinical Psychology, 39*(4), 371–382.

First, M. B., Frances, A., & Pincus, H. A. (2002). *DSM-IV-TR handbook of differential diagnosis*. American Psychiatric Publishing Inc.

Gersh, E., Hallford, D. J., Rice, S. M., Kazantzis, N., Gersh, H., Gersh, B., et al. (2017). Systematic review and meta-analysis of dropout rates in individual psychotherapy for generalize anxiety disorder. *Journal of Anxiety Disorders, 52*, 25–33.

Goddard, E., Wingrove, J., & Moran, P. (2015). The impact of comorbid personality difficulties on response to IAPT treatment for depression and anxiety. *Behavioral Research and Therapy, 73*, 1–7.

Goldstein-Piekarski, A. N., Williams, L. M., & Humphreys, K. (2016). A trans-diagnostic review of anxiety disorder comorbidity and the impact of multiple exclusion criteria on studying clinical outcomes in anxiety disorders. *Translational Psychiatry*. https://doi.org/10.1038/tp.2016.108

Hayes, A. M., Laurenceau, J. P., Feldman, G., Strauss, J. L., & Cardaciotto, L. A. (2007). Change is not always linear: The study of nonlinear and discontinuous patterns of change in psychotherapy. *Clinical Psychology Review, 27*(6), 715–723.

Koelen, J. A., Luyten, P., Eurelings-Bontekoe, L. H., Diguer, L., Vermote, R., Lowyck, B. et al. (2012). The impact of level of personality organization on treatment response: A systematic review. *Psychiatry*, *75*(4), 355–374.

Lecrubier, Y. (1998). The impact of comorbidity on the treatment of panic disorder. *Journal of Clinical Psychology*, *8*, 11–14.

Links, P. S., Shah, R., & Eynan, R. (2017). Psychotherapy for borderline personality disorder: Progress and remaining challenges. *Current Psychiatry Reports*. https://doi 10.1007/s11920-017-0766-x

Mohr, D. C., Beutler, L. E., Engle, D., Shoham-Salomon, V., Bergan, J., Kaszniak, A. W., et al. (1990). Identification of patients at risk for nonresponse and negative outcome in psychotherapy. *Journal of Consulting and Clinical Psychology*, *58*(5), 622–628.

Newman, M. G., Przeworski, A., Fisher, A. J., & Borkovec, T. D. (2010). Diagnostic comorbidity in adults with generalized anxiety disorder: Impact of comorbidity on psychotherapy outcome and impact of psychotherapy on comorbid diagnoses. *Behavioral Therapy*, *41*(1), 59–72.

Olatunji, B. O., Broman-Fulks, J. J., Bergman, S. M., Green, B. A., & Zlomke, K. R. (2010a). A taxometric investigation of the latent structure of worry: Dimensionality and associations with depression, anxiety, and stress. *Behavioral Therapy*, *41*(2), 212–228.

Olatunji, B. O., Cisler, J. M., & Tolin, D. F. (2010b). A meta-analysis of the influence of comorbidity on treatment outcome in the anxiety disorders. *Clinical Psychology Review*, *30*(6), 642–654.

Ollendick, T. H., Jarrett, M. A., Grills-Taquechel, A. E., Hovey, L. D., & Wolff, J. C. (2008). Comorbidity as a predictor and moderator of treatment outcome in youth with anxiety, affective, attention deficit/hyperactivity disorder, and oppositional/conduct disorders. *Clinical Psychology Review*, *28*(8), 1447–1471.

Reuter, L., Munder, T., Altmann, U., Hartmann, U., Strauss, B., & Scheidt, C. E. (2016). Pretreatment and process predictors of nonresponse at different stages of inpatient psychotherapy. *Psychotherapy Research*, *26*(4), 410–424.

Sanatinia, R., Wang, D., Tyrer, P., Tyer, H., Crawford, M., Cooper, S., et al. (2016). Impact of personality status on the outcomes and cost of cognitive-behavioural therapy for health anxiety. *British Journal of Psychiatry*, *209*(3), 244–250.

Shea, M. T., Widiger, T. A., & Klein, M. H. (1992). Comorbidity of personality disorders and depression: Implications for treatment. *Journal of Consulting and Clinical Psychology*, *60*(6), 857–868.

Siegfried, N. (1998). A review of comorbidity: Major mental illness and problematic substance use. *Australia and New Zealand Journal of Psychiatry*, *32*(5), 707–717.

Van Bronswijk, S. C., Lemmens, L. H., Viechtbauer, W., Huibers, M. J., Antz, A., & Peeters, F. P. (2018). The impact of personality disorder pathology on the effectiveness of cognitive therapy and interpersonal psychotherapy for major depressive disorder. *Journal of Affective Disorders*, *225*, 530–538.

Walczak, M., Ollendick, T., Ryan, S., & Esbjorn, B. H. (2018). Does comorbidity predict poorer treatment outcome in pediatric anxiety disorders? An updated 10-year review. *Clinical Psychology Review*, *60*, 45–61.

World Health Organization. (1992). *The ICD-10 classification of mental and behavioral disorders: Clinical descriptions and diagnostic guidelines*. World Health Organization.

World Health Organization. (2022). *The ICD-11 classification of mental and behavioral disorders: Clinical descriptions and diagnostic guidelines*. World Health Organization.

Chapter 6

RESISTANCE AND NONCOMPLIANCE

Opposition to psychotherapy or some aspect of it transpires with resistance and noncompliance. The opposition can be subtle or more overt, but blocks progression. As mentioned in the Preface, resistance and noncompliance are quite negative terms, and I do not believe that this type of problem accounts for most instances of failure to progress in psychotherapy, but it is a definite impediment for some clients. A sizeable percentage of the literature pertaining to poor outcomes in psychotherapy does focus on resistance and noncompliance. We will look at what the literature has to say about this topic and then turn to key sources of opposition.

The literature includes various terms such as resistance, noncompliance, nonresponse, and ambivalence, with the first three at least, often used interchangeably. Nonresponse is not ideal, as there can be multiple factors accounting for this occurrence beyond client opposition. One factor that we have looked at is severity of mental illness (see the Complexity chapter) that does impede psychotherapy progress. Examining extreme nonresponse in cognitive therapy for depression, Coffman et al. (2007) found that severity in regard to intensity and persistence of symptoms, functionality, and primary support, accounted for the poor outcomes. Focusing on inpatients (576) with depression, anxiety, adjustment problems, and eating disorders, Melchior et al. (2016) discovered that nonresponse occurred with 11% of the inpatients, and was linked to dysfunction in terms of low education level, non-employment, and chronicity of the given illness. Hence, nonresponse is different than resistance and noncompliance, and arises from severe illness manifestations and dysfunction. Interestingly, nonresponse appears more likely when clients have low subjective distress, probably because there is limited motivation (Mohr et al., 1990; Reuter et al., 2016).

Resistance and noncompliance imply a negative stance toward psychotherapy on the part of the client. Beutler et al. (2002) indicate that despite many differences, there is an assumption that resistance (and noncompliance) is both a dispositional trait and an in-therapy state of oppositional, angry, irritable, and suspicious behaviors, that bodes poorly for treatment effectiveness. Beutler et al. (2002) view reactance as an extreme form of resistance capturing

DOI: 10.4324/b23346-7

its dimensional nature. A meta-analysis of 13 controlled studies involving 1,208 patients, looked at the relationship between the approach taken by the therapist in terms of directive and non-directive and degree of client reactance: high reactance participants had better outcomes when the therapist took a non-directive approach, rather than a directive and more authoritarian stance (Beutler et al., 2018a). This is actually quite intuitive because psychotherapy typically does not work well with a highly directive (authoritarian) stance, since it is a collaboration, and for a client who is highly resistant such an approach would be like rubbing salt in an open wound. Interestingly, though, Beutler et al. (2018a) also found that for some psychotherapy participants with high reactance, a very directive stance worked better. In an earlier meta-analysis of 12 studies involving 1,102 participants, Beutler et al. (2011) ascertained that those with low levels of trait-like resistance responded better to directive types of treatment, whereas individuals with high levels of such resistance improved more with nondirective treatments.

Shifting focus somewhat, Beutler et al. (2018b) examined coping style in terms of externalizing (deal with change outwardly) and internalizing (deal with change by looking inwardly), and a treatment-symptom versus insight focus, updating the 2011 meta-analysis. They found that a treatment-symptom focus is more effective for externalizing patients, whereas an insight focus works well for those who internalize. There is an intuitive logic to this as those who are introverted with a tendency to internalize would seem to value insight more, and those with an extroverted personality who externalize might value insights to a lesser extent and focus more on the treatment and symptoms. The idea here being that matching internalizing and externalizing styles to treatment-symptom or insight focus can potentially reduce resistance and improve progress.

Resistance and noncompliance can apply to various aspects of psychotherapy including: recognition of feelings, fantasy, and motives; feelings toward the therapist; demonstration of self-sufficiency; reluctance to change behaviors; reaction to limited therapist empathy and support (Messer, 2002). This type of reaction to therapy is more likely to transpire when prerequisites for psychotherapeutic change are not in place, with these consisting of: sense of necessity, willingness to experience anxiety or difficulty, awareness of the problem, confronting the problem, effort, hope, and social support (Hanna, 1996). Working with the client to address any potential limitations pertaining to these prerequisites can help to reduce resistance and noncompliance. Relevant to the role of social support is a study of 46 clients and 19 therapists partaking in long-term therapy, finding that insecure client attachment to the therapist was linked to resistance, and understandably secure attachment correlated with low resistance (Yotsidi et al., 2018). Facilitating secure attachment is the therapist reaction to any client resistance, because if negative it can impair the relationship (Newman, 2002). Hence, it is important for therapists to be aware of their own reaction to client resistance and address it therapeutically, such as exploring the reasons for why resistance is emerging, instead of responding with negative emotions conveyed in facial expressions. If therapists are to work with client resistance they must recognize it, and this appears to be easier than what might seem to be the case, based on a study comparing resistance during analytically oriented and behavioral therapy: Verhulst and van de Vijver (1990) found that despite very different forms of therapy, both types of therapists agreed that avoiding and fighting behaviors were the most prominent expressions of resistance and also that therapists' questions regarding the nature and origin of the client's complaints were a common trigger.

Opposition as a defensive response constitutes another theme in the literature (Bernstein & Landaiche, 1992; Rowe, 1996). Self-psychology views resistances as protecting a vulnerable self, designed to maintain levels of organization achieved within the context of traumatic or challenging life circumstances (Rowe, 1996). Consistent with a defensive motivation, client resistance increases when the therapeutic setting is not viewed as safe, and decreases when therapists provide a safe framework (Bernstein & Landaiche, 1992). The defense perspective contrasts with the typical notion of resistances being only interferences to progress that must be overcome (Bernstein & Landaiche, 1992; Rowe, 1996). In the Personality Disorders chapter, we looked at how these disorders represent extreme and enduring expressions of normal defensive processes, and in the case of Narcissistic Personality Disorder, the grandiose aspect is a defensive compensation for vulnerabilities. It does follow that oppositional behavior in psychotherapy can serve as a defense against vulnerability, even if not narcissistic. Tapping into the notion of defense of vulnerabilities, is the "wounded self" concept, capable of producing resistance when the wound is threatened (Dowd, 2016).

A more positive reframing of resistance and noncompliance is ambivalence, the notion being that conflicting thoughts, emotions, goals, and motivations produce oppositional behavior. Unlike in the mathematical realm, opposites in the psychological realm do not cancel each other out: plus 3 and minus 3 do not cancel to 0, but instead coexist producing an ambivalent state of mind. Highly relevant is the concept of cognitive dissonance: when opposing cognitions exist, an unpleasant psychological state known as cognitive dissonance arises, typically motivating behavior to resolve the inconsistency. Dissonance can produce irritable, angry, and oppositional behavior, at least until it is resolved. For example, "I care deeply about my family," and "My drinking behavior is harming my family." These cognitions are clearly inconsistent and produce an unpleasant psychological state (dissonance). Ideally, by making a client aware of the inconsistency, motivation for psychotherapy progress will ensue: "I do care about my family and can't deny that my drinking is hurting them, so I do need to alter my drinking behavior." However, what happens if this shift to resolution does not occur? If the person is aware of the inconsistency, the answer is often negative emotions flowing from dissonance, including irritability and anger producing oppositional behavior. For example, "What the hell does that therapist know. He is such a nerd, he probably has never tied one on and let loose." Another option is to psychologically bury the inconsistency by dissociating from it, which is hard to do if the therapist is bringing it up as with motivational interviewing interventions, in which case anger and opposition is more likely, assuming the client fails to work with the problem.

Taking the perspective that some ambivalence is inevitable in psychotherapy and can impede progress, Shaffer and Simoneau (2001) suggest that "exercising" ambivalence to strengthen tolerance for it is helpful. Resistance can be reduced allowing the client to be more open to a wider range of change options. A value of this perspective is that even though the ideal with motivational interviewing approaches is for the client to become aware of inconsistencies and respond with increased motivation for change, in practice this does not always occur, and even if there is increased motivation fear of change can be overwhelming, at least until the client has progressed with psychotherapy. Inducing greater tolerance for ambivalence, while not negating the informational and motivational value, would seemingly reduce opposition to psychotherapy, thereby facilitating its progression. Resistance has been viewed as an expression of ambivalence (Arkowitz & Engle, 2007; Urmanche et al., 2019), and if this is the case, then resolving or "exercising" ambivalence can almost certainly reduce resistance.

Now that we have an understanding of what the literature says about resistance, noncompliance, nonresponse, and ambivalence, we will consider key sources of resistance and noncompliance, including emotional, dysfunctional patterns of behavior, and personality factors. A major source of resistance and noncompliance is transference, or more precisely negative transference, since positive transference can actually facilitate progress. Given the power of transference in psychotherapy outcomes, we will examine it separately in the Transference chapter, but keep in mind that negative transference can produce oppositional behavior.

EMOTIONAL

Emotions are highly relevant to psychotherapy, and certain ones such as fear, anger, shame, and guilt can produce resistance. Fear often results in inhibition and avoidance, the latter challenging to overcome, and particularly so when it reaches the intensity and persistence of Avoidant Personality Disorder. Anger is another powerful emotion when it comes to blocking progress with therapy. Nicholas provides an example of both emotions. This young engineer showed quite a bit of anger toward his parents and sister during the assessment. He discussed how his parents held fearful perspectives regarding the world, telling him and his sister how it is impossible to get ahead, and only family can be trusted. They led a simple life with his father working for the same company over decades and his mother mostly staying at home. Nicholas was angry that his sister "sided" with them and did not advance, only holding a fairly menial job and continuing to live with their parents. He claimed that no one in the family respected his educational accomplishment, and instead seemed to perceive a threat in that he was leaving them behind. He reported this as traumatic as he was looking for support. Demonstrating fear and avoidance like his parents and sister, he avoided romances and reported that his limited efforts did not work as women found him to be too intense in his views. He also avoided any challenging job remaining at a low level.

Over approximately a year we worked on Nicholas's issues from both an emotional and cognitive perspective, looking at how his parents and sister perceived multiple threats eliciting fear and communicated this to him. He learned how their world view instilled fear, that in turn reinforced the world view, with both fostering avoidance. We also looked at the anger he felt at the violation of not being supported and praised. Although he seemed to progress well with the understanding, perhaps not surprising given his intelligence, it became apparent that he was stuck because of the fear and anger. He would not progress to a romance rationalizing why he could not, nor could he let go of the anger toward his parents and sister blaming them for virtually everything. When I attempted to confront this resistance to change, he would become angry and reiterate the issues with his family. We looked at transference issues, but this approach was not effective. Eventually therapy ended with his fear and anger remaining fixed. Consistent with a self-psychology perspective, Nicholas's fear based avoidance and anger could be interpreted as a defense to keep him safe from challenges, but might also be viewed as a block to overcome from a more traditional perspective on resistance. Regardless of the purpose served, he was extremely resistant to relinquishing it, thereby not advancing beyond some insight.

Shame and guilt are emotions also capable of blocking progress. David was in his 40s when seen, the assessment revealing depression connected with shame and guilt regarding his mother, who had always been very supportive and caring. He was from South Africa, and as a Caucasian decided it was best to move to Canada when the Apartheid era ended. Every year he visited his mother, and this seemed to relieve his negative feelings about leaving her behind, at least when combined with regular phone calls. The real problem began when she started to show signs of dementia, at which point his sense of shame and guilt escalated, and also sadness as he now realized that he was really losing her. He wanted to move back but realized that this would not be feasible given his great job and family in Canada. As his mother's cognitive functioning deteriorated his shame and guilt worsened and depression set in. I started an antidepressant and provided psychotherapy. We looked at how with shame and guilt there is a perception at some level of a social error, and he certainly felt he was a bad person for abandoning her there. I attempted to reframe his perspective to instead of being "bad" he actually is a very caring person and doing everything feasible, as with paying for her nursing home and a personal attendant. We also went over limits and boundaries we all have to accept, meaning he could not move back to South Africa, nor would his mother benefit from moving to Canada as this would worsen her disorientation. Furthermore, she did not want to leave South Africa in the first place. It was clear that he was very self-punitive and we worked on self-support, but he persisted in beating himself up about the situation such that progress was limited, mostly consisting of less sadness and depression aided by the antidepressant.

These two client examples, with fear and anger in the first and shame and guilt in the second, come to mind as the most intense when it comes to resistance derived from emotional sources. Less intense variants are common, and both the therapist and client need to consider them.

Therapist Role

The starting point is to appreciate how powerful negative emotions can be in blocking progress in therapy. Pay particular attention to fear, anger, shame, and guilt, as these emotions can generate resistance. Working with the emotion information processing aspect (see the Expectations chapter) is crucial, because it provides an understanding of what the client is experiencing and ways to remedy the problem. Fear occurs in response to the unconscious or conscious perception of threat or danger, anger violation or damage, and shame social (and perhaps moral) transgression with guilt likely a variant. Altering the relevant perceptions can moderate the intensity of these emotions: reduced perceptions of threat/danger, violation/damage, and social transgression will settle fear, anger, and shame/guilt, respectively. In the case of shame and guilt, the client is likely very self-critical, and a shift to self-acceptance is crucial (see the Impaired States and Processes for Mental Health chapter). The therapist provides a role model, as with acknowledging mistakes and not reacting negatively to flaws the client demonstrates. I go over how mistakes are unavoidable given that no one is perfect, and instead of blaming learn from them. Fostering shifts to positive emotions via perceptions of gains (happiness) and reward potential (interest), further diminishes the intensity of the negative emotions.

Client Role

As with the therapist, embrace the notion of emotion information processing, as this provides a straightforward guide to working with emotions like fear, anger, and shame/guilt. Realize that although there is a logical aspect to emotion information processing, perception is a critical aspect: emotions are based on perceptions of core circumstances and not absolute reality. Experiencing the emotion, it might seem as if the feeling is fully justified, but by simply altering the perception, the emotion shifts. For example, "This exam coming up is going to be way too difficult," triggering fear. Altering the perception to, "The exam is manageable and a chance for me to show my knowledge and advance," replaces fear with positive feelings. Work with the therapist, and also on your own, to shift emotion information in a positive direction. Regarding being self-critical, we live in a very blame oriented society, but within the spirit of perceptions and not absolute reality, there is no objective reason for why this is so. Quite the contrary, since no one is perfect mistakes will happen and learning from them instead of berating yourself is more fitting. Such an approach fosters self-acceptance which favors positive emotions and enhanced resilience.

DYSFUNCTIONAL PATTERNS OF BEHAVIOR

The term, dysfunctional, suggests that these patterns of behavior can and often will produce resistance blocking progress with psychotherapy. One such pattern noted in the above section is being self-critical. From the therapist's perspective, it almost seems like these clients have passed a life sentence on themselves to ensure continual suffering, as with David feeling never-ending shame and guilt over his mother remaining in South Africa. David only had to relinquish this self-punishment and be open to the possibility that he was doing everything possible given the obvious constraints.

There are numerous variations on the theme of dysfunctional patterns of behavior producing resistance. Sandra provides an interesting example related to maintaining excessive weight. Extreme thought distortions qualifying as psychosis was a key feature, with Sandra developing a delusion that a boss wanted her beyond the work relationship. She began to interpret his actions as supporting a romance, and the actions of other work colleagues as attempting to sabotage this occurrence. As is often the case with such belief systems there was some truth, based on her boss being flirtatious and charismatic. However, there was no evidence he was prepared to have an affair with her. The distorted perspective triggered a crisis when she confronted some of the suspected adversaries at a party. She ended up having to go on disability and begin treatment. During her teenage years, she was of fairly normal weight, but due to a medical condition began gaining weight. Prior to significant weight gain she was sexually assaulted at a party, and this trauma made her fearful of sexual advances by men. She found that as her weight went up interest from men went down, producing a feeling of safety. When I entered the picture, she was very overweight and in her late 30s. Excessive weight is a major risk factor for several diseases and she developed diabetes. We worked on her fears and the trauma experience, including losses and pain derived from it, and how as a woman she has the power to resist the advances of men, excessive weight not required to achieve this. However, her weight advanced to the point where she developed heart failure and had to be placed in an induced coma to survive. When she left the hospital (fortunately) I reiterated an early suggestion to have bariatric surgery, as it would deal with the weight problem and possibly her various health issues. Despite learning to normalize her psychotic level perceptions pertaining to her now former boss, she persisted in the sense that weight is ironically safer for her and repeatedly rejected the notion of surgery. The dysfunctional behavior of weight gain and the supporting belief system remained quite fixed impeding progress. In the Motivation chapter, we considered Hank under the related notion of rigid patterns of behavior, who persisted in a pattern of distrust and deceptions to the point where he lost his career, home, and therapist, with a move away from Toronto being necessary. Numerous efforts on my part failed to work, because the dysfunctional pattern was too engrained and virtually guaranteed failure to progress in both life and therapy.

Dysfunctional patterns of behavior frequently arise from two sources: non-traumatic and traumatic repetitive maladaptive behavior (Bowins, 2010). Regarding the former, there appears to be a capacity derived from human evolution for learning patterns of behavior from caregivers, in that patterns of behavior demonstrated by members of one's hunting-gathering group were adaptive for the given environment (Bowins, 2010). In such a setting with exposure to a substantial number of individuals, deviant patterns would probably have been opposed or diluted. However, outside of this evolutionary context that characterized approximately 95–99% of our evolution, a child is often exposed to only two or even one caregiver, providing a scenario where dysfunctional patterns can be dominant. For example, avoidance, excessive aggression, and self-criticisms. In the case of David, his father was a very critical person both of himself and others, providing a template for self-criticism that David internalized. These patterns of behavior are a default option arising with triggering circumstances, such as any challenging scenario. To replace such patterns of behavior with more functional ones, the client has to consciously overlearn the alternative pattern of behavior, applying it whenever and wherever possible. Eventually, with repetition it will become the default option. For instance, a person with an aggressive response pattern has to consciously practice restraint and more thoughtful responses, and self-critical people such as David have to practice self-support.

As pertains to trauma-based repetitive maladaptive behavior, the problem is the dissociated fragmented nature of the experience. Therapists, researchers, and clients often focus on "forgotten" aspects of trauma, but what is really occurring is that the various emotional and cognitive aspects are dissociated, repeating as fragments interfering with adequate mental processing. Regarding memory, recall is best when an experience is comprehensively processed such that it represents an intact mental event, but this does not transpire when the emotional and cognitive aspects of the experience are dissociated. With trauma, fusion of the various emotional and cognitive aspects of the event is often too painful or overwhelming at a conscious level, producing defensive dissociation of these components, and consequently, their repetition as fragments (Bowins, 2010). Hence, an emotional response or behavior can repeat as it is disconnected, as with Sandra's fear of sexual assault that instead of being processed and resolved, remained unresolved instilling an ongoing dysfunctional motivation for weight gain. The nature of this type of emotion and response pattern insulates it from modification with changing circumstances. Activating the grieving process helps to resolve it, because every trauma involves losses of some form, and in contrast to the trauma based dissociation of emotions and cognitions, grieving these losses assists in fusing the emotional and cognitive aspects of the traumatic experience. A technique that can assist with healthy grieving is writing comprehensive and positive narratives relevant to the traumatic event, because it addresses the dissociated elements and fuses them in a constructive fashion. Unfortunately, as is evident from Sandra's example, going back in time to facilitate fusion with grieving, and techniques fostering it, does not always work ideally.

Even though dysfunctional patterns are very challenging, there are ways that therapists and clients can approach them.

Therapist Role

Attempt to identify dysfunctional patterns of behavior which can take time. Appreciate the origins of such behavior, with them often arising from either a learning experience early in life or trauma related (Bowins, 2010). The distinction is important because in the instance of internalized patterns of behavior, the key strategy involves unlearning the dysfunctional pattern by having the client consciously overlearn the more functional alternative. David, for example, needed to practice self-understanding and praise of his own actions ongoing to replace the intense self-critical pattern with one of self-acceptance. Hank needed to practice being open and trusting in any reasonable circumstances for psychotherapy to progress. If the dysfunctional pattern of behavior is trauma based, then efforts to fuse the dissociated cognitive and emotional aspects of the traumatic experience are important. Reactivating (or activating) grieving pertaining to losses related to the trauma helps achieve this fusion. Encouraging the client to generate positive and complete narratives relevant to the traumatic event can assist with healthy grieving.

Client Role

If the dysfunctional pattern of behavior is derived from exposure to the given pattern early in life, realize that by consciously overlearning the alternative option/s whenever and wherever feasible via practice, you can replace dysfunctional behavior with much more adaptive behavior. Eventually the new more adaptive behavioral pattern will become a habit form of memory and your default option. If the dysfunctional pattern of behavior is related to trauma, appreciate that it is often linked to dissociated emotion and thought aspects of the trauma. Without fusion these dissociated elements persist, and the only way to manage them is to strive for fusion, which is advanced by activating or reactivating the grieving process based on losses associated with the trauma. When people talk of working through traumatic experiences, I believe that this is what is transpiring with a goal of fusing the dissociated elements.

Making the effort to generate narratives pertaining to the traumatic event that reframe the occurrence in a meaningful way helps with grieving.

PERSONALITY FACTORS

In the Personality Disorders chapter, we looked at how more extreme and enduring expressions of normal defensive processes produce these problems, and how within the personality disorder range, more severe variants impede psychotherapy. In some instances this failure to progress arises from compromised functioning: avoiding anything stressful including positive change with intense Avoidant Personality Disorder, precarious grandiose compensation for vulnerabilities in Narcissistic Personality Disorder, inability to function independently with Dependent Personality Disorder, too fixed and repetitive defensive containment of anxiety in Obsessive-Compulsive Personality Disorder, and dysfunctional overuse of immature defense mechanisms with Borderline Personality Disorder.

Personality disorder based failure to progress in psychotherapy can also involve more direct resistance and noncompliance. This occurrence is frequently seen with Narcissistic Personality Disorder when the vulnerabilities are touched, given that they are like an open physical wound, the slightest contact producing a negative reaction. Severe vulnerabilities foster intense compensation—the grandiose aspect—and this can be and often is abrasive with no empathy and consideration for others, including the therapist. With severe Avoidant Personality Disorder and Dependent Personality Disorder, attempts to have the client approach rather than avoid and reduce dependency can be perceived as both a threat and violation, producing fear and anger, respectively. However, given their anxiety it might be expressed in a passive aggressive form, such as not attending or showing up to a session very late. Attempts to alter very rutted compulsive behavior not uncommonly trigger overt resistance, blocking progress with Obsessive-Compulsive Personality Disorder. Given the underlying normal personality trait of conscientiousness, which appears to predispose the client to this personality disorder, they usually attend punctually but resist efforts to modify the compulsive behavior. In the case of Borderline Personality Disorder, expression of immature defenses including acting out, splitting, and idealization and devaluation (at least the latter part), express intense resistance and noncompliance.

In addition to personality disorder sources of resistance and noncompliance, certain normal personality traits can be involved. Normal personality dimensions include extraversion-introversion, neurotic-emotionally stable, open-closed to experience, agreeable-antagonism, and conscientious-negligence (Costa & McCrae, 1992). As presented in the Personality Disorders chapter, neurotic-emotionally stable really is reactivity giving it a meaningful evolutionary context. Extreme reactivity predisposes to various mental health problems, and certainly Borderline Personality Disorder when an individual has been traumatized early in life, not surprising given the damaging nature of trauma that is greatly amplified with high reactivity. Intense reactivity can also produce resistance and noncompliance. Early in the chapter we looked at how reactance as an extreme form of resistance impedes psychotherapy progress (Beutler et al., 2011, 2018a). Highly reactive individuals are likely to respond negatively to even relatively benign psychotherapy interventions, perceiving them as a threat and/or violation producing resistance.

One of my clients, Hamid, provides a striking example of extreme reactivity. Now middle-aged he worked in the insurance sector at a fairly junior level, not advancing largely because any occurrence he viewed as negative produced an intense response. Eventually he was laid off, and has never secured anything other than marginal employment, instead relying on family members for financial support. In the romance sphere, he has not sustained a long-term relationship, other than one when very young. Friendships have not persisted because when he perceives any behavior reflecting adversely on him, he reacts with anger and confronts the person. His level of reactivity is something to behold, even with antidepressant medication to reduce anxiety. Real progress in therapy, beyond improving his mood and self-concept, was very difficult to achieve, and we shifted to infrequent medication and supportive therapy sessions. One time when he was running low on medication, he called me to renew his prescription. Unfortunately, his chosen pharmacy was not all that functional (95% of my problems with prescribing arise from 5% of pharmacies), and the phone just kept ringing. Eventually that day, at the end of the week, I got through and left a clear message for a renewal. Returning after the weekend I was besieged by several exasperated and angry messages from Hamid regarding no prescription, despite him still having some pills left, and the option of his pharmacy covering him until they got hold of me. I called Hamid and during the conversation expressed how this is an example of reactivity that limits him. He exploded denying any fault on his part, including reactivity. I was only able to calm him when I explained that some pharmacies do not work ideally, at which point he shifted the anger to them. It turned out that the pharmacy did get my message but the person he spoke to was not aware of this. Hamid's level of reactivity is off the charts so to speak, translating into resistance with any therapeutic input that can even remotely be interpreted as negative, to his obvious detriment.

The agreeable-antagonism dimension, which might be better labeled agreeable-disagreeable, produces resistance and noncompliance when the person has a high degree on the adversarial side. One mid-30s client, Brendon, provides such an example. He works in the technology sector, and like Hamid at a junior level with failure to progress in regard to career, romances, or friendships. The problem for Brendon is that he is very disagreeable and prone to see violations or damaging intent or behavior. Interpretations, and even comments that would be readily agreed with by other clients, have produced negative responses that are very obvious. His facial expression clouds over, body becomes tense, and he either remains deathly silent or expresses resentment for the comment. Addressing his silence prompts him to express the anger. Any intervention that can be interpreted as anything other than supportive meets with resistance (disagreeable/antagonism), very clearly limiting progress with therapy. One time he presented a muscle related problem, the cause evident given my early general medical practice work, and to help him I ventured a comment on what the problem is and solution. At times, I cannot help providing this input and some of my referral sources send me clients with comorbid medical conditions, being aware of my early career general medicine experience. True to disagreeable form, Brendon reacted negatively expressing how I should not be giving such input, because even though it aligned with what his physiotherapist explained the solution did not. It was only when I shifted to how hard it must be for him to work with the pain that the clouds of disagreement cleared. I have worked on his issue from an emotional information perspective, going over how perceptions of violation and damage, often independent of any objective reality, trigger anger. He claims that his perceptions align with reality. Transference interpretations have also been presented eliciting a disagreeable response. Unfortunately, his level of antagonism is so extreme that significant progress with psychotherapy, and life for that matter, is very unlikely.

Extreme levels on the negative side of the normal personality dimensions of neurotic-emotionally stable (reactivity) and agreeable-antagonism produce resistance and noncompliance, and both are very difficult for the therapist and client to work with.

Therapist Role

Based on my experience, and I am confident that of other therapists, extreme reactivity and antagonism (disagreeable) are very challenging to make any real headway with, and therapy usually does not go beyond supportive and/or medication interventions. In some instances, the client will be open to how reactivity or being disagreeable impairs them. Having the client provide examples of people they know who are very reactive or contrary, antagonistic, and disagreeable, might help with insight into their personality. However, the notion that they have a detrimental personality feature will often be strongly reacted to and/or disagreed with. It is important to note that some people have high levels of both reactivity and antagonism, with the combination almost certainly a deal breaker for psychotherapy progress. With one or both of these personality traits, my earlier suggestion for therapists to be self-supportive comes into play, as despite your best efforts strong resistance is likely. Avoid getting angry and reacting strongly, easier said than done, because this just provides a model for reacting and being antagonistic, reinforcing their personality traits. For possible techniques see the Clients Role.

Client Role

The client has more impact than the therapist in this instance, because if you persist in being extremely reactive and/or disagreeable psychotherapy will not progress well. The best strategy is to have a one-to-one talk between your personality and rational side to decide which option is best: persist with repeated failures and limited progress in life, or accept the problem and work on it with the help of a therapist. If option one is selected, which occurs by default if you deny that any personality issue is involved, then psychotherapy is not recommended. If you take option two, appreciate that while it is not feasible to change fundamental features of personality, you do have the capacity to override inclinations derived from these personality traits, and this process gets easier with more practice. For example, in the case of extreme reactivity I have clients suppress (a mature defense mechanism) their immediate response, apply balanced thought, and with this input respond. I refer to this as SUPPRESS-THINK-RESPOND. Outcomes are far better than with unfiltered reacting. In the case of antagonism, apply a correction factor, appreciating that you lean to the disagreeable side based on perspectives of violation and damage, which can be corrected by shifting in the opposite direction. Consider the analogy of a marksman (or woman) firing eight degrees to the left reaching the target by correcting eight degrees to the right. An awareness that perceptions of violation and damage trigger anger is crucial. It is also important to realize that personality derived responses and outcomes reinforce each other: intense reactivity and/or antagonism alienates people who withdraw, and this response on their part produces reactive and disagreeable behavior, leading to further isolation.

SUMMARY NOTE

Resistance and noncompliance are different than nonresponse that can arise from issues such as how severe a given mental illness is. With resistance and noncompliance there is a dispositional aspect and also negative expression in therapy. While this behavior can be viewed as largely confrontational, it can also be seen as a defensive response serving a self-protective function. Ambivalence and cognitive dissonance play a role, with options of either resolving the dissonance or fostering more tolerance of ambivalence to facilitate progress in psychotherapy. Major sources of resistance and noncompliance consist of negative transference (covered in a separate chapter), emotional, dysfunctional patterns of behavior, and personality factors. Regarding emotional sources, fear, anger, shame and guilt stand out, because when these emotions are strong intense resistance often transpires. Dysfunctional patterns of behavior come in many forms, such as a pattern of being highly self-critical, sharing a common endpoint of generating resistance to positive change with psychotherapy. Personality factors both in terms of personality disorders and select normal traits—intense reactivity and antagonism/disagreeable—produce pronounced resistance. Despite the very negative connotations of resistance and noncompliance for progress with psychotherapy, by working with ambivalence, negative emotions, dysfunctional patterns of behavior, and personality factors, there is much that the therapist and client can do to move therapy ahead.

REFERENCES

Arkowitz, H., & Engle, D. (2007). Understanding and working with resistant ambivalence in psychotherapy: An integrated approach. In S. G. Hoffman & J. Weinberger (Eds.), *The art and science of psychotherapy* (pp. 171–188). Routledge.

Bernstein, P. M., & Landaiche, N. M. (1992). Resistance, counterresistance, and balance: A framework for managing the experience of impasse in psychotherapy. *Journal of Contemporary Psychotherapy, 22,* 5–19.

Beutler, L. E., Edwards, C. J., & Someah, K. (2018a). Adapting psychotherapy to reactance level: A meta-analytic review. *Journal of Clinical Psychology, 74*(11), 1952–1963.

Beutler, L. E., Harwood, T. M., Michelson, A., Song, X., & Holman, J. (2011). Resistance/reactance level. *Journal of Clinical Psychology, 67*(2), 133–142.

Beutler, L. E., Kimpara, S., Edwards, C. J., & Miller, K. D. (2018b). Fitting psychotherapy to patient coping style: A meta-analysis. *Journal of Clinical Psychology, 74*(11), 1980–1995.

Beutler, L. E., Moleiro, C., & Talebi, H. (2002). Resistance in psychotherapy: What conclusions are supported by research. *Journal of Clinical Psychology, 58*(2), 207–217.

Bowins, B. E. (2010). Repetitive maladaptive behavior: Beyond repetition compulsion. *American Journal of Psychoanalysis, 70,* 282–298.

Coffman, S. J., Martell, C. R., Dimidjian, S., Gallop, R., & Hollon, S. D. (2007). Extreme nonresponse in cognitive therapy: Can behavioral activation succeed where cognitive therapy fails? *Journal of Consulting and Clinical Psychology, 75*(4), 531–541.

Costa, P. T., & McCrae, R. R. (1992). *Revised NEO personality (NEO-PI-R) and NEO five factor inventory (NEO-FFI) professional journal manual.* Psychological Assessment Resources.

Dowd, E. T. (2016). Resistance and the wounded self: Self-protection in service of the ego. *American Journal of Clinical Hypnosis, 59*(1), 100–113.

Hanna, F. J. (1996). Precursors of change: Pivotal points of involvement and resistance in psychotherapy. *Journal of Psychotherapy Integration, 6*(3), 227–264.

Melchior, H., Schulz, H., Kriston, L., Hergert, A., Hofreuter-Gatgens, K., Bergelt, C., et al. (2016). Symptom change trajectories during inpatient psychotherapy in routine care and their associations with long-term outcomes. *Psychiatry Research, 238,* 228–235.

Messer, S. B. (2002). A psychodynamic perspective on resistance in psychotherapy: Vive la resistance. *Journal of Clinical Psychology.* https://doi: 10.1002/jclp.1139

Mohr, D. C., Beutler, L. E., Engle, D., Shoham-Salomon, V., Bergan, J., Kaszniak, A. W., et al. (1990). Identification of patients at risk for nonresponse and negative outcome in psychotherapy. *Journal of Consulting and Clinical Psychology, 58*(5), 622–628.

Newman, C. F. (2002). A cognitive perspective on resistance in psychotherapy. *Journal of Clinical Psychology.* https://doi: 10.1002/jclp.1140

Reuter, L., Munder, T., Altmann, U., Hartmann, U., Strauss, B., & Scheidt, C. E. (2016). Pretreatment and process predictors of nonresponse at different stages of inpatient psychotherapy. *Psychotherapy Research, 26*(4), 410–424.

Rowe, C. E. Jr. (1996). The concept of resistance in self psychology. *American Journal of Psychotherapy, 50*(1), 66–74.

Shaffer, H. J., & Simoneau, G. (2001). Reducing resistance and denial by exercising ambivalence during the treatment of addiction. *Journal of Substance Abuse Treatment, 20*(1), 99–105.

Urmanche, A. A., Oliveira, J. T., Goncalves, M. M., Eubanks, C. F., & Muran, J. C. (2019). Ambivalence, resistance, and alliance ruptures in psychotherapy: It's complicated. *Psychoanalytic Psychology, 36*(2), 139–147.

Verhulst, J. C., & van de Vijver, J. R. (1990). Resistance during psychotherapy and behavior therapy. *Behavior Modification.* https://doi.org/10.1177/01454455900142004

Yotsidi, V., Stalikas, A., Pezirkianidis, C., & Pouloudi, M. (2018). The relationships between client resistance and attachment to therapist in psychotherapy. *Journal of Contemporary Psychotherapy, 49*, 99–109.

Chapter 7

IMPAIRED STATES AND PROCESS FOR MENTAL HEALTH

Mental health is characterized by key states and processes consisting of: activity, psychological defense mechanisms, social connectedness, psychological regulation, human specific cognition, self-acceptance, and adaptability (Bowins, 2021). Intact functioning on these states and processes equates with mental health, including positive affectivity over negative affectivity, while impaired functioning produces mental illness (Bowins, 2021). Psychotherapy actually appears to work by advancing these states and processes for mental health, with both strategies specific to a type of therapy and non-specific factors playing a role (Bowins, 2021). An across therapy (often referred to as trans-therapy, not to be confused with trans-gender therapy) approach to enhancing the effectiveness of psychotherapy, consists of applying the most robust specific and non-specific strategies for advancing the key states and processes for mental health (Bowins, 2021). This across therapy option is particularly important given the seemingly endless increase in the number of specific forms of psychotherapy, that has created confusion for psychotherapists, students, consumers, funders, and teaching institutions. Space limitations prevent an extensive coverage of these key states and processes for mental health and their actual and potential role in psychotherapy, but interested readers can consult *States and Processes for Mental Health: Advancing Psychotherapy Effectiveness* (Bowins, 2021). From the perspective of our current focus on barriers to psychotherapy progress, impairments to each of the states and processes for mental health serve as limiting influences. For each state and process a brief description of its role in mental health and illness will be presented, followed by how impairments impede psychotherapy progress.

ACTIVITY

Human evolution in hunting-gathering groups ensured that we had to be active searching for food, safe resting and sleeping places, and other resources, in contrast to our tree dwelling higher primate relatives who are quite fine with limited activity (Pontzer, 2017; Raichlen & Alexander, 2017). Highly relevant are the Behavioral Approach/Activation System (BAS) and Behavioral

DOI: 10.4324/b23346-8

Inhibition System (BIS), with the former approach and activation focused generating reinforcement, and the BIS system withdrawal and inhibition oriented consistent with a lack of reinforcement and punishment (Fowles, 1988; Gray, 1987). Solid activity aligns with a profile of high BAS and low BIS. Various mental illnesses including anxiety and depression arise when there is high BIS, and low BAS also occurs with depression (low BAS/high BIS) (Bowins, 2021). Hypomania consists of low BIS and high BAS, and I have proposed that it can override depressive inhibition to a large extent by reversing the depressive profile of high BIS and low BAS (Bowins, 2008). Hypomania is also effective in managing anxiety, because it shifts the high inhibition (elevated BIS) of anxiety to low inhibition (Bowins, 2008). Templates exist for override mechanisms, and of great relevance for BIS and BAS, physiological and emotional states such as intense hunger, thirst, and anger, can override behavioral inhibition (Cosmides & Tooby, 2000). By encouraging a client to be very active a therapist is actually inducing hypomania of a sort (Bowins, 2008). Clinicians who fear this scenario might want to consider that hypomania as a personality equivalent—hyperthymic temperament—confers ongoing resilience to depression (Akiskal & Pinto, 1999).

As pertains to psychotherapy, strategies such as behavioral activation diminish BIS and enhance BAS, increasing activity and reducing depression and anxiety (Bowins, 2021). This is a major reason why behavioral activation is across therapy and trans-diagnostic (across specific mental illnesses) process, although it is typically viewed as a behavioral therapy strategy. Generally, activity of various forms—physical, social, nature, cognitive (for cognitive health), art/hobby, and music—counters mental illness and advances mental wellbeing in the general population (Bowins, 2020).

Given the power of activity for mental health, and role of high BIS and low BAS in mental illness, it follows that restricted activity with high BIS and low BAS can impede progress in psychotherapy. Inhibited behavior (high BIS) translates into the client not acting on material worked on during psychotherapy sessions, and what transpires between sessions is crucial. If a client just discusses issues and does not enact any change, then real progress beyond insight is greatly limited or non-existent. Every psychotherapist has experienced clients who do not act on any of the insights or techniques acquired and remain essentially unchanged. A major reason for this is inhibited behavior, with the most dramatic manifestation Avoidant Personality Disorder characterized by massive inhibition. Low BAS also plays a role in lack of change, and particularly when depression is present, expressed as little motivation, energy, and effort to advance. The combination of high BIS and low BAS can greatly impede positive change during psychotherapy.

Other than for those practicing behavioral activation therapy, the notion of focusing on activity might seem unusual, but I have noted that therapists working from many different orientations suggest physical, social, mental, and other forms of activity to clients, highlighting the role of activity in mental health.

Appreciate that by altering high BIS, and also low BAS, anxiety and depression will diminish, and material worked on in psychotherapy sessions will be transformed into real change, an occurrence that is very pleasing for psychotherapists to see. Behavioral activation mostly entails having the client approach rewarding scenarios in a graded way, from least to most challenging, to overcome fear and avoidance. The reward increases BAS and further reduces BIS. Securing rewards favors positive emotions such as happiness and interest over negative emotions. Assisting behavioral activation work is a focus on emotional information processing. As covered in the Expectations chapter, fear occurs when cognitive activating appraisals detect threat or danger, and sadness loss. These emotions can be amplified by thought processes resulting in excessive fear/anxiety and sadness/depression. By altering the perceptions to see less in the way of threat/danger and loss, fear and sadness can be reduced. This change in emotional information processing favors reduced BIS and increased BAS, transforming inhibition into activation. Real progress in therapy is then more likely to transpire. Encourage and support clients in being active in as many safe and rewarding ways as is viable. Keep in mind that instead of the client waiting for the right emotional state, act first and then experience the benefit.

PSYCHOLOGICAL DEFENSE MECHANISMS

Much as the immune system protects us against pathogens, psychological defense mechanisms shield us from emotional stressors. The notion of psychological defense mechanisms originated with Sigmund Freud, who along with his daughter, Anna, identified specific mechanisms and their characteristics including: major means of managing conflict and disturbing affect, relatively unconscious, discrete from one another, reversible despite being the hallmark of major psychiatric syndromes, adaptive as well as pathological (Freud, 1949). In more recent times, Vaillant (1994) described the maturity level of psychological defense mechanisms, referring to both the adaptive value of the defense and the age when it is most likely to be expressed. Based on this system, classical psychological defense mechanisms consist of (Freud, 1949; Vaillant, 1994):

Immature: splitting, idealization and devaluation, projection, hypochondriasis, somatization, undoing, acting out, schizoid fantasy, and denial.
Intermediate/neurotic: intellectualization, rationalization, repression, isolation, reaction formation, displacement, and dissociation.
Mature: humor, sublimation, anticipation, altruism, and suppression.

This arrangement suggests that there are discrete categories—immature, intermediate/neurotic, mature—and as has been mentioned, we prefer discrete entities to simplify information processing. However, they are continuous from immature to mature, as revealed by Trijsburg et al. (2000) who had experienced psychoanalysts rate the maturity level of classical psychological defense mechanisms, and then applied various statistical analyses to the data including factor analysis. A unidimensional representation from least to most mature emerged.

My research enters the picture at this point, with a model of psychological defense mechanisms involving two major templates: positive cognitive distortions and dissociation (Bowins, 2004, 2006). Regarding the former, reality is elusive and our perspectives naturally represent distortions, either positive or negative. Depression and anxiety are characterized by negative distortions, with excessive loss oriented perspectives in the former, and threat and danger in the case of anxiety (Beck, 1991; Beck & Clark, 1997). The evolution of human intelligence has amplified sadness, fear, and other emotions, by making the underlying cognitive appraisals more intensive, extensive, and with a temporal component (Bowins, 2004, 2006). Consequently, we are vulnerable to intense negative emotions. I proposed that psychological defense mechanisms evolved to diminish negative emotions and bolster positive ones (Bowins, 2004, 2006). Positive cognitive distortions place a self-enhancing and upbeat spin on events, and hence, favor positive emotions. Good mental health is distorting experience to enhance the self and provide a positivity bias, while diminishing negativity (Beck, 1991; Beck & Clark, 1997). Consistent with how natural events are organized continuously, the positive cognitive distortion defense capacity ranges from mild to extreme. Mild versions enable people to slightly alter their perceptions of various experiences by placing a positive, self-enhancing spin on them so that they are less negative and threatening, with hope being one of the most powerful. Moderate level expressions involve more extensive cognitive distortions, consisting of excessive fantasy involvement, magical thinking, and over-valued ideas. Extreme cognitive distortions cross into the realm of delusions not consistent with reality. Psychotic cognitions are then at the extreme end of a cognitive distortion continuum (Kingdon & Turkington, 1994; Landa et al., 2006).

The second proposed major psychological defense mechanism template of dissociation has a history longer than that of classical defense mechanisms. There is a range of perspectives pertaining to this involved entity. Some researchers such as Janet view it as a breakdown or disruption in the usually integrated functions of consciousness (in Marmar et al., 1994; Putman, 1985). Dissociation has also been viewed as a positive defensive process, such as by Watkins and Watkins (1997), who see it as a natural organizing principle of the psyche giving humans the ability to adapt, think, act, and respond. Freud (1895/1964) indicated that dissociation can dislocate affect from ideas, while Vaillant (1977) suggests that dissociation permits the ego to so alter the internal state that the pain of conflict seems irrelevant. I interpret dissociation as the ability to detach from adverse emotional states and circumstances, providing a key psychological defense mechanism template (Bowins, 2004, 2012).

Detaching from negative emotions favors positive emotions. According to this model, dissociation ranges from mild-extreme along a continuum (Bowins, 2004, 2012):

Mild: emotional numbing, absorption in positive foci, and compartmentalization.
Moderate: depersonalization and derealization.
Extreme: amnesia and identity fragmentation.

In regard to impeded progress in psychotherapy, psychological defense mechanism functioning is very important to consider. In the Personality Disorders chapter, we noted how immature classical defense mechanisms often block or substantially impede progress with psychotherapy, and how this frequently transpires with Borderline Personality Disorder. Responding to psychotherapeutic interventions with acting out, idealization/devaluation, splitting, and the like, makes real progress a challenge. We also noted how improvement of this personality disorder always entails a shift from immature to mature defenses. While personality disorders, and in particular Borderline Personality Disorder, is the most extreme example of immature classical psychological defense mechanisms impeding progress, any instance of these defenses expressed in therapy can slow progress.

In the case of cognitive distortions, negative ones favoring depression and anxiety, typically impede psychotherapy because they induce behavioral inhibition: loss focused perspectives reduce hope limiting behavioral activation, and threat/danger cognitions directly inhibit actions. With reduced behavioral activation and increased behavioral inhibition, there is less potential for actual change with psychotherapy. Dissociation also plays a role because when extensive, such that the person is detached from feeling states and adverse events in their life, there is less chance that the client will successfully process these feelings and experiences. Clients who are emotionally detached from others including their partner and the therapist, usually do not advance these relationships until they connect with their feelings. Fortunately, steps can be taken to remedy defense mechanism manifestations that limit psychotherapy progress.

Therapists must note any immature classical defenses and actively address them as covered in the Personality Disorders chapter. Demonstrating to clients how the given immature defense impairs functioning while mature ones enhance coping capacity is very helpful, because mature defenses can be consciously learned and practiced. Negative cognitive distortions are the norm with depression and anxiety, and are generally pervasive in mental illness. By diminishing behavioral activation and intensifying behavioral inhibition, negative cognitive distortions impede progress with mental illness and psychotherapy. Identifying and addressing these distortions, and facilitating a shift to positive ones emphasizing hope and the potential to succeed, help ensure progress.

If a client appears dissociated from feelings, events, and relationships, assisting the person in connecting with them by working through any emotional pain will facilitate progress, because although being dissociated reduces stress, it can block progression with the given mental health issue and psychotherapy. If dissociation is more intense as a response to trauma, address it as covered in the Resistance and Noncompliance chapter, which essentially involves attempts to fuse the dissociated emotional and cognitive aspects of the traumatic experience, with a useful strategy consisting of reactivating (or activating) the grieving process by identifying losses associated with the traumatic occurrence, aided by positive comprehensive self-narratives. Negativity is present in everyone's life, and applying milder dissociation in terms of absorption in positive foci and compartmentalization helps clients cope with adversity, without incurring the limitations of more intense dissociation. Hence, guiding clients in the use of these two forms of dissociation is encouraged.

SOCIAL CONNECTEDNESS

The vast majority of human evolution has been within a social context consisting of hunting-gathering groups. Consequently, we have a social brain ensuring that we view the world in social terms and rely on others. While some alone time is pleasant, as a persistent state of affairs this usually translates into loneliness and mental health problems. Quality counts, though, and negative social contact such as bullying can be very damaging. The term social connectedness refers to positive social contact, a key influence in good mental health. Impaired social connectedness is usually thought of as loneliness and isolation with these terms often applied synonymously. However, there is a distinction, as a person can be on their own and not feel lonely, and also with others and feel lonely. This occurrence highlights the importance of perception and feeling connected: a person can be with others and feel lonely due to not feeling a connection, and on their own but feel connected to a segment of society. Loneliness is linked to worse mental health, such as indicated by suicidal behavior. Stickley and Koyanagi (2016) assessed 7,403 households with the Adult Psychiatric Morbidity Survey and Clinical Interview Schedule Revised. Loneliness was associated with suicidal behavior (ideation and attempts), and participants reporting the most severe degree of loneliness had a 3.45 greater odds ratio for lifetime suicide attempts, and 17.37 greater odds ratio for past year suicide attempts, even when conditions like depression were taken into account.

Social connectedness has a powerful impact on psychotherapy progress, largely due to the role it plays in the therapeutic alliance, which will be covered in the chapter of that name in the Interactive Influences section. Clients with a capacity to socially connect are more likely to bond to their therapist, ushering in all the benefits that the therapeutic alliance produces. On the other hand, a person who has trouble connecting with others will struggle to form a solid therapeutic alliance to the detriment of progress in psychotherapy. The implications of this will be looked at in more detail in the Therapeutic Alliance chapter, but various aspects such as responding constructively to transference interpretations, internalizing positive thoughts and behavior demonstrated by the therapist, and accepting suggestions are impacted negatively.

To improve social connectedness, assess the client's social history pertaining to friendships and romances. A history characterized by disconnection usually indicates an insecure attachment style, often confirmed by their early life with caregivers. When this scenario is detected appreciate that both the therapeutic relationship and the client's interactions with others will be challenged. From these two related occurrences, progress with psychotherapy is likely to be impeded. There are various ways of working on the therapeutic relationship that will be covered in the Therapeutic Alliance chapter, but it is often helpful to address the client's early life circumstances with caregivers, and how this has influenced trust and the capacity to form relationships with others, potentially including the therapist. This sets the stage for managing issues in the therapeutic relationship, and also problems they report in relationships outside of therapy. Such is the potency of a good therapeutic alliance that any client factor impacting negatively on it necessitates being focused on.

PSYCHOLOGICAL REGULATION

Biological processes ranging from the cellular to ecosystem level rely on regulation, an occurrence that also applies to psychological processes. When psychological regulation is impaired, mental illnesses including depression, anxiety, eating disorders, personality disorders, psychosis, and mania, are more likely to occur (Bowins, 2021). Top-down regulation is often involved, referring to higher cortical processes and structures, such as the prefrontal cortex, exerting control over limbic system and paralimbic structures. In the case of depression and anxiety impaired top-down regulation is strongly implicated. Regarding depression, studies based on neuroimaging reveal excessive activation of limbic and other emotion-related structures, and attenuated activity of frontal regions involved in emotion regulation (Arnsten, 2009, 2011; Beauregard et al., 2006). Beauregard et al. (2006) found that compared to non-depressed controls, depressed subjects demonstrated impaired down-regulation of sad feelings, ensuring that they had difficulty containing depression-related emotions.

As pertains to anxiety, amplified activity in limbic and paralimbic structures, and decreased activity in the prefrontal cortex has been reliably found (Delgado et al., 2006; Hartley & Phelps, 2010; Larson et al., 2006), a pattern interpreted as the prefrontal cortex failing to exert sufficient top-down regulation of limbic system fear/anxiety responses (Arnsten, 2009, 2011; Hartley & Phelps, 2010; Larson et al., 2006). A negative feedback loop appears to transpire with both anxiety and depression, whereby with sufficient stress the regulatory function of the prefrontal cortex is impaired, resulting in excessive negative emotional responses that generate additional stress, further impairing prefrontal cortex regulation, and so on and so forth (Arnsten, 2009, 2011). The mutually reinforcing negative emotion and thought cycles covered in the Reinforcement Parameters chapter, also challenge regulatory capacity. Deficient emotion regulation results in excessive negative emotions, whereas robust regulation fosters positive emotions. Regarding vulnerability to depression and anxiety, a predisposition to excessive limbic system activity, at least for negative emotions, and/or deficient regulation over this activity is implicated, with stress bringing out the vulnerability and worsening it. Depression and anxiety are tightly linked to emotions, with amplified sadness fostering depression and amplified fear anxiety, the amplification necessitating emotion regulation while also making it challenging (Bowins, 2004, 2006).

Regulation problems extend to psychosis and mania (Bowins, 2008, 2011). Psychosis consists of extreme variants of thought content (delusions), thought form, and sensory-perceptual experiences (hallucinations). There is a range on these cognitive parameters from highly reality congruent characterizing normal states to reality incongruent, the latter psychosis. An important question consists of, why is it that we typically do not experience more extreme versions in the conscious and awake state? A related question is, why do we experience psychotic equivalents when dreaming including bizarre ideation, loose thought form, and sensory-perceptual experiences not at all reality based? The answer I came up with is that to facilitate reality congruency, necessary for adaptive functioning and hence evolutionary fitness, extreme variants of these cognitive events have to be regulated out of the conscious and awake state (Bowins, 2011, 2016). During sleep when we are inactive, and hence, do not have to be reality congruent, extreme variants do not require regulation and are expressed as psychotic equivalents. Psychosis in the conscious and awake state arises when the regulatory processes over thought content, thought form, and sensory-perceptual experiences are impaired. For greater detail, evidence backing this assertion, and what transpires with schizophrenia and other manifestations of psychosis see Bowins (2011, 2016).

Mania also appears to involve impairments to regulation. Under the Activity section of this chapter, I presented my theory regarding hypomania as a depressive (and anxiety) override defense mechanism, reducing behavioral inhibition (BIS) and enhancing behavioral activation (BAS) (Bowins, 2008). In contrast to hypomania which is adaptive, mania is typically not due to excess energy expenditure that is usually unproductive, reduced sleep, impaired control of sexual and aggressive urges, out of control thought processes, and psychosis. I have proposed that mania arises due to impaired regulation of the hypomania defense, removing the brakes so to speak (Bowins, 2008, 2016). Many instances of hypomania progressing to mania involve substance use/abuse and/or antidepressants, both capable of impairing regulation over hypomania. The common comorbidity of psychosis likewise implicates regulation deficits, not surprising given that events capable of fostering the conversion of hypomania to mania, could also impair regulation over thought content, thought form, and sensory-perceptual processes. For a detailed coverage of this topic including the role of neural connectivity and dysconnectivity, see Bowins (2016).

Robust psychological regulation over emotions and other mental illness events favors good mental health, while impaired regulation produces mental illness of various forms. When it comes to psychotherapy progress, regulation impairments create problems both in terms of more severe manifestations of mental illness, and from this more challenge in remedying the problem (see the Complexity chapter), and also the direct impact on psychotherapy. For instance, too intense negative emotions including fear/anxiety, sadness, anger, guilt, and shame can impede progress with psychotherapy, because it is difficult for the client to progress beyond the emotional reaction. In addition to emotions, intense cognitive distortions can block psychotherapy progress. We looked at how psychosis represents extreme thought content, thought form, and sensory-perceptual experiences. Below the realm of psychosis resides excessive fantasy involvement, magical thinking, and over-valued ideas. For example, many people hold ideas pertaining to conspiracy theories and racial beliefs that are not quite at the level of psychosis, but close. If a client holds such beliefs and progress with therapy depends on the person relinquishing the belief/s, then progress is impaired.

Based on the notion of regulation there are strategies to moderate excessive emotions and overly intense beliefs, thereby facilitating progress with mental health issues and psychotherapy. As pertains to excessively intense emotions, there are emotion regulation strategies that a therapist can employ. At various points, we have looked at emotion information processing and how cognitive activating appraisals with certain core themes trigger the emotion. By addressing the information aspect of negative emotions, therapists have a powerful method of reducing the intensity to moderate or low levels, and shifting the client to positive emotions. If there is excessive sadness focus on perceptions of loss by having the client identify all losses perceived. Then work on adjusting perceptions that are not fully warranted, and shifting to a focus on gains and successes. Too intense fear/anxiety entails strong perceptions of threat and danger. Help the client distinguish the landscape and separate objective from only subjective threats in order to moderate fear. Emphasizing reward and interesting aspects of challenges, helps to replace threat and danger perceptions producing fear, with positive thoughts favoring happiness and interest. In the case of anger, work on perceptions of violation and damage by having the client generate alternative perspectives. By working with emotion information processing intense negative emotions can be moderated and even replaced with positive emotions.

When it comes to extreme thought distortions including those at a psychotic level, the cognitive behavioral approach of normalization is the most optimal strategy to bring the distortions back to a more moderate level (Kingdon & Turkington, 1994; Landa et al., 2006). The first step is to provide evidence.

Ask the client for supporting evidence that will hold out in court. Rarely if ever can the person provide evidence, let alone any of this quality. The next step is to generate alternative perspectives to their preferred one, treating their view as one hypothesis and not challenging it. The more alternatives that the person can generate, the more diluted the severely distorted one becomes. The individual also shifts to greater openness and flexibility furthering perspective shifts. The third strategy is to test alternative perspectives if feasible, as this strategy will usually confirm a less intense option than the one the person has favored. If the distortions are clearly in the psychotic realm, normalization can be advanced by antipsychotic medication.

The strategies outlined for normalizing extreme emotions and thoughts have the theme of regulation, and I have suggested that many strategies therapists employ actually comprise cognitive regulatory control therapies, given that they act by enhancing regulation (Bowins, 2013). Therapists can increase their effectiveness in managing excessive negative emotions and distorted cognitions by conceptualizing the approach as regulation based, and employing normalizing strategies that follow from this understanding.

HUMAN SPECIFIC COGNITION

Various cognitive processes operating at an unconscious level characterize humans, hence the term "human specific cognition" (Bowins, 2011, 2016; Burns, 2009; Fiszdon et al., 2007). The term is not meant to imply characteristics entirely absent in other species, as traits are derived from preexisting templates due to how natural selection conserves resources by building on what has come before (Darwin, 1959). It instead refers to the compilation of cognitive abilities that distinguish us behaviorally from other species. These include basic cognition, social cognition, and motivational states. Basic cognition largely refers to executive functions including: working memory, initiation, inhibition, cognitive flexibility, task completion, attention, planning, organizing, and monitoring (Gross & Grossman, 2010). Broader basic cognitive capacities like problem solving, the ability to generalize, and overall intelligence rely extensively on executive functions. Social cognition includes how people think about themselves, others, social situations and interactions (so-called Theory of Mind capacities), plus emotional information processing, understanding complex social-emotional scenarios such as irony and sarcasm, and social drive limitations (Combs et al., 2013; Fiszdon et al., 2007; Rapp et al., 2014). Motivation comes in various forms, such as striving for knowledge, self-improvement, self-actualization, career accomplishments, friends, romantic partners, and more basic needs such as food, water, and shelter (Mahurin et al., 1998).

Solid functioning intellectually, socially, and behaviorally follows from intact basic cognition, social cognition, and motivation. Impairments comprising so-called negative symptoms result in mental health problems including: Autism Spectrum Disorder, Intellectual Disability, Attention Deficit Hyperactivity Disorder (ADHD), Schizophrenia, Bipolar Disorder I (mania) (Ancin et al., 2013; Owen, 2012; Purper-Ouakil & Franc, 2011; Waltereit et al., 2014). Human specific cognition relies on intact neural connectivity, and dysconnectivity underlies negative symptoms (Bowins, 2016). Regulation also relies on intact neural connectivity, and the extensive neural dysconnectivity associated with the negative symptoms of schizophrenia and Bipolar I (mania) appears to impair regulation over psychotic level cognitions and containment of hypomania to an adaptive level, resulting in psychosis and mania, respectively (Bowins, 2016). The role of neural connectivity and dysconnectivity in mental health and illness is a fascinating, but complex, topic covered extensively in the Negative Symptom chapter of my book, *Mental Illness Defined: Continuums, Regulation and Defense* (Bowins, 2016).

The focus here is on impediments to progress in psychotherapy, and negative symptoms play a significant and largely hidden role, consistent with how their contribution to mental illness is often not well recognized. At a general level, extensive negative symptoms make the mental illness more severe creating difficulties in managing the problem. Additionally, negative symptoms are challenging to treat, although currently this is a hotly debated topic in part due to the commercialization of therapeutic programs. More specific to psychotherapy, deficits to human specific cognition translate into difficulty working with the cognitive, social, and motivational demands of treatment. Impairments to executive functions, such as working memory, cognitive flexibility, and attention, make it challenging for the client to process information, including transference interpretations, and even working hypothesis of mental illness issues. Social cognitive impairments limit a person's ability to respond appropriately to the social interaction between therapist and client, thereby interfering with the therapeutic alliance. These deficits also make it difficult to transform any social learning into constructive improvements in social interactions with others. When it comes to motivational states, deficits block or reduce the transformation of therapeutic interventions into behavioral advances away from therapy. Understanding how negative amotivational symptoms, even in those not suffering from schizophrenia or severe mood disorders, play a role in this outcome can reduce the frustration experienced by therapists when the client fails to progress.

Appreciating human specific cognition and negative symptoms also fosters ways to effectively intervene. The starting point is an awareness and understanding of negative symptoms, an occurrence that is not usual due to how deemphasized human specific cognition and negative symptoms are in mental health and illness. However, given the extent of basic cognition, social cognition, and motivation, we all have specific deficits, it really being how many and to what extent, and how they interfere with healthy functioning relevant to mental health. As pertains to basic cognitive deficits, which mostly consist of executive functions (working memory, initiation, inhibition, cognitive flexibility, task completion, attention, planning, organizing, and monitoring), therapists can get an approximate idea of the client's level of functioning by how the person processes information and approaches tasks in therapy sessions, even during the assessment. Can the person inhibit one stream of thought and flexibly shift to another? Is the individual able to remain focused on a given topic? Does the person demonstrate organization and initiation? Thinking in terms of these executive functions and evaluating the client's behavior relevant to them, provides approximations that will improve with practice. If pronounced executive functioning deficits are discovered then information might have to be parsed out in smaller units, and kept in concrete terms with more examples provided. Language will also have to be kept quite basic. The client might have to be redirected back to topics if attention is an issue.

In regard to social cognitive deficits, descriptions provided by the client of their relationships, and also therapy interactions, help identify limitations. Strategies including more extensive role-playing and assistance in identifying emotions in facial expressions (facial expression recognition) are helpful. Components of complex social interaction such as irony, sarcasm, and even humor, are elusive when a person has significant social cognitive impairments, and these might have to be explained and distinguished by repeat examples. When basic motivation is impaired targeting specific behavioral improvements, as opposed to more general motivation, can help a client progress with behaviors outside of psychotherapy. For instance, focus on having a person telephone old friends, instead of trying to advance socialization in general. While psychotherapists might find working with negative symptoms to be unfamiliar and challenging, it can be very rewarding to see the client progress in terms of these issues, and even more when the gains in human specific cognition transform into further psychotherapy gains.

SELF-ACCEPTANCE

Believing in yourself and being self-supportive foster good mental health, whereas not accepting who you are and being self-critical favor mental illness. Self-esteem refers to a person's global appraisal of his/her positive or negative value, based on evaluations in more specific areas, and is equivalent to self-regard, self-estimation, and self-worth (Mann et al., 2004). Low self-esteem contributes to internalizing forms of mental illness such as depression, anxiety, eating disorders, and psychosis: studies of a longitudinal design have found that low self-esteem from childhood to early adulthood is a predictor of later depression and anxiety (Ginsburg et al., 1998; Isomaa et al., 2013; Trzesniewski et al., 2006). Externalizing mental health problems including aggression, antisocial behavior, and school problems are linked to low self-esteem, at least for younger people (Donnellan et al., 2005; Jessor et al., 1998). Whereas low self-esteem appears to favor mental illness, high self-esteem fosters mental health (Jones & Heaven, 1998; Rouse, 1998).

Self-concept and self-efficacy represent perspectives pertaining to oneself, with self-concept the sum of an individual's beliefs and knowledge regarding personal attributes and qualities, being equivalent to self-image and self-perception, whereas self-efficacy refers to beliefs regarding specific behaviors such as math ability (Mann et al., 2004). Negative self-concept links with mental illnesses such as depression and suicidal tendencies, while positive self-concept is associated with good mental health (Andersson et al., 2014; Mann et al., 2004). Andersson et al. (2014) conducted a cross-sectional study of 3,981 adults, finding that those with low global self-efficacy (self-concept) were more likely to suffer from mental illness than those with high global self-efficacy.

Self-esteem and self-concept, and hence self-acceptance, strongly influence psychotherapy progress. Generally, very low self-esteem and self-concept translate into greater severity of a given condition, given the link between these psychological constructs and various forms of mental illness. As we covered in the Complexity chapter, severity of mental illness can be a limiting factor for progress in psychotherapy. Specific to psychotherapy, low self-acceptance diminishes confidence in making changes required for progress. For instance, if a client greatly doubts their social skills they might not make the effort to build friendships or romances. Likewise, when a client lacks confidence in their academic ability, the person is less likely to seek work retraining opportunities. The low confidence arising from poor self-esteem and/or self-concept is reinforced by the failure to progress: with no or an inadequate effort to change due to low confidence their life remains unchanged, strengthening the low confidence.

Self-criticisms comprise another way that poor self-acceptance limits progress in psychotherapy, and constitutes one of the most potent impediments there is! Many people seeking psychotherapy have a self-critical nature. I rarely encounter a client who is very self-accepting with robust self-esteem and self-concept, and this scenario often occurs in the context of the client's life going well until a major loss transpires producing depression. Life, including psychotherapy progress, usually involves a certain number of steps back for every few steps forward, with progress steps forward > steps backward. A self-critical nature adds steps backward to any challenging endeavor, often translating into more steps backwards than forwards, contributing heavily to low self-esteem and self-concept. It is then very important for therapists to determine if and to what extent the client is self-critical. Allowing the person to talk openly about events in their life usually reveals this aspect of their nature. If not, then you can simply ask the client if they tend to be harsh on themselves. Once you determine that a client is self-critical realize that the person will typically have low self-esteem and self-concept, due to the ongoing negative self-evaluations and self-perspectives. Poor self-acceptance will limit the client's progress. To intervene both overt and modeling approaches apply. I discuss with the client how they limit their progress in life by being self-critical, usually applying the analogy: "It is like a home builder who adds bricks but then uses a sledge hammer against the foundation." This analogy fits well and sometimes gets a smile or knowing nod. Then I add, "Would it not make more sense for the home builder to put down the sledge hammer and just add more bricks?" A rhetorical question, but something that is unfamiliar to self-critical people. I cover how we live in a blame oriented society where mistakes have to be accounted for and punished. I mention that everyone makes mistakes, including me as a therapist, and what counts is learning from the mistakes to reduce the likelihood of a repetition. When the client starts criticizing some action during a session, I request that they stop the self-punishment and determine what can be learned. Therapists also help self-critical clients by modeling supportive behavior, both toward the client and their own self. If the client makes a mistake such as showing up late, rather than assigning blame go over what can be learned and applied to future visits, such as taking into account public transportation delays and arriving 15 minutes early.

ADAPTABILITY

Organisms have to adapt to their environment to survive and thrive. This applies to people and the circumstances they encounter each day. Higher functioning people automatically adjust behavior to fit with changing circumstances, and given that the only constant is change, this is an ongoing process. Low functioning people usually apply behavior that does not align with the circumstances encountered. Adaptability entails two major components, consisting of the capacity to engage in actions and fitting behavior to circumstances (Bowins, 2021). The first component is easy to miss, but is crucial, because a person must act to adapt. Inadequate actions can arise from behavioral inhibition exceeding behavioral activation (BIS > BAS). Inadequate activity can also follow from negative symptoms, including impaired basic cognition, social cognition, and motivation, with the latter highly significant. Fitting behavior to circumstances is facilitated by intact human specific cognition and behavioral activation over behavioral inhibition, but also requires ongoing flexibility that entails neural plasticity. The neural representation of behavior is known as Hebbian plasticity, with the well quoted saying that "neurons that fire together wire together" (Power & Schlaggar, 2016). When behavior results in certain neurons firing together that behavior is represented at a neural level, and the more repetition the more robust the wiring (Power & Schlaggar, 2016). Neural representation of behaviors facilitates future adaptive responses for the particular circumstances, providing a template for responding that can be modified for novel scenarios. On the other hand, reduced neural plasticity compromises adaptability, and evidence reveals that this occurrence is linked to mental illness: Waltereit et al. (2014) provides research support for impaired neural plasticity in Autism Spectrum Disorder (ASD), mental retardation (Intellectual Disability), and schizophrenia. Intact neural plasticity facilitates adaptation to changing circumstances.

When it comes to progress in psychotherapy, reduced neural plasticity, behavioral inhibition exceeding behavioral activation, and negative symptoms will be limiting factors. Another key limiting factor is repetitive maladaptive behavior. Every therapist has encountered clients who maintain the same maladaptive approach to changing circumstances resulting in ongoing setbacks. Consistent with this scenario, psychotherapy progress is limited and positive change does not transpire. Noting this occurrence, Albert Ellis founded Rational Emotive Therapy designed to target rigid behavior patterns (Ellis, 1980). Given how fixed and repetitive these patterns are, assertive and even aggressive confrontation was applied (Ellis, 1980). When a client relinquishes a dysfunctional pattern of behavior, and adopts a flexible approach adapting behavior to circumstances, both psychotherapy and their life progress.

Even though it can be challenging to foster adaptive behavior there are approaches that will help. As a therapist, detect repetitive maladaptive patterns of behavior and address these with the client. Distinguish if the pattern is traumatic or non-traumatic in nature. If trauma related, approach it as covered under Psychological Defense Mechanisms. For non-traumatic patterns the client must overlearn adaptive alternatives to the dysfunctional pattern by applying such behavior wherever and whenever feasible. Appreciate that repetitive maladaptive behavior is challenging to change and needs to be worked on over several sessions, often with assertive re-direction to the issue. The reward for both the client and therapist is real change of the sort Albert Ellis sought. If limited adaptability arises from behavioral inhibition exceeding behavioral activation, then apply the behavioral activation strategies presented in the Activity section. Negative symptoms impairing adaptability can be addressed as described in the Human Specific Cognition section. Ultimately, the goal is to improve neural plasticity and the capacity to adapt to ever changing circumstances. I have noted that clients demonstrating maladaptive patterns of behavior, and more generally failing to demonstrate adaptive actions, often take an either/or perspective such as good/bad, right/wrong, succeed/fail. Shifting this type of perspective to adaptive/maladaptive fosters a more flexible approach, with an obvious emphasis on adjusting behavior to circumstances.

SUMMARY NOTE

States and processes for mental health—activity, psychological defense mechanisms, social connectedness, psychological regulation, human specific cognition, self-acceptance, and adaptability—facilitate progress with psychotherapy when robust, and hinder it when there are impairments. Understanding these states and processes and applying the strategies outlined will foster progress with both psychotherapy and the client's mental health issues, with mutual reinforcement transpiring: as psychotherapy progresses the client's mental illness/s will recede, fostering further and often faster progress in psychotherapy, more mental health gains, and so on and so forth. As an added advantage, positive affectivity over negative affectivity follows from the states and processes for mental health, such as with behavioral activation securing rewards producing positive emotional responses, psychological defense mechanisms favoring positive emotions over negative ones, and emotion regulation diminishing negative emotions on an ongoing basis.

REFERENCES

Akiskal, H., & Pinto, O. (1999). The evolving bipolar spectrum: Prototypes I, II, III, and IV. *Psychiatric Clinics of North America*, *22*, 517–534.

Ancin, I., Cabranes, J. A., Santos, J. L., Sanchez-Moria, E., & Barabash, A. (2013). Executive deficits: A continuum schizophrenia-bipolar disorder or specific to schizophrenia? *Psychiatry Research*, *47*(11), 1564–1571.

Andersson, L. M., Moore, C. D., Hensing, G., Krantz, G., & Staland-Nyman, C. (2014). General self-efficacy and its relationship to self-reported mental illness and barriers to care: A general population study. *Community Mental Health*, *50*(6), 721–728.

Arnsten, A. (2009). Stress signaling pathways that impair prefrontal cortex structure and function. *Nature Reviews Neuroscience*, *10*, 410–422.

Arnsten, A. (2011). Prefrontal cortical network connections: Key sites of vulnerability in stress and schizophrenia. *International Journal of Developmental Neuroscience*, *29*(3), 215–223.

Beauregard, M., Paquette, V., & Levesque, J. (2006). Dysfunction in the neural circuitry of emotional self-regulation in major depressive disorder. *Neuroreport*, *17*(8), 843–846.

Beck, A. (1991). Cognitive therapy: A 30-year retrospective. *American Psychologist*, *46*(4), 368–375.

Beck, A., & Clark, D. (1997). An information processing model of anxiety: Automatic and strategic processes. *Behavior Research and Therapy*, *35*(1), 49–58.

Bowins, B. (2008). Hypomania: A depressive inhibition override defense mechanism. *Journal of Affective Disorders*, *109*, 221–232.

Bowins, B. E. (2011). A cognitive regulatory control model of schizophrenia. *Brain Research Bulletin*, *85*, 36–41.

Bowins, B. E. (2004). Psychological defense mechanisms: A new perspective. *American Journal of Psychoanalysis*, *64*, 1–26.

Bowins, B. E. (2006). How psychiatric treatments can enhance psychological defense mechanisms. *American Journal of Psychoanalysis*, *66*, 173–194.

Bowins, B. E. (2012). Therapeutic dissociation: Compartmentalization & absorption. *Counselling Psychology Quarterly*, *25*(1), 307–317.

Bowins, B. E. (2013). Cognitive regulatory control therapies. *American Journal of Psychotherapy*, *67*(3), 215–236.

Bowins, B. E. (2016). *Mental illness defined: Continuums, regulation, and defense*. Routledge.

Bowins, B. E. (2020). *Activity for mental health*. Academic Press.

Bowins, B. E. (2021). *States and processes for mental health: Advancing psychotherapy effectiveness*. Academic Press.

Burns, J. K. (2009). Reconciling 'the new epidemiology' with an evolutionary genetic basis for schizophrenia. *Medical Hypothesis*, *72*, 353–358.

Combs, D. R., Finn, J. A., Wohlfahrt, W., Penn, D. L., & Basso, M. R. (2013). Social cognition and social functioning in nonclinical paranoia. *Cognitive Neuropsychiatry*, *18*(6), 531–548.

Cosmides, L., & Tooby, J. (2000). Evolutionary psychology and the emotions. In M. Lewis & J. Haviland-Jones (Eds.), *Handbook of emotions* (2nd ed., pp. 91–115). The Guilford Press.

Darwin, C. (1859). *On the origin of species*. Signet Classic. (Original work published 1858.)

Delgado, M. R., Olsson, A., & Phelps, E. A. (2006). Extending animal models of fear conditioning to humans. *Biological Psychology, 73*(1), 39–48.

Donnellan, M. B., Trzesniewski, K. H., Robins, R. W., Moffitt, T. E., & Caspi, A. (2005). Low self-esteem is related to aggression, antisocial behavior, and delinquency. *Psychological Science, 16*(4), 328–335.

Ellis, A. (1980). Rational-emotive therapy and cognitive behavior therapy: Similarities and differences. *Cognitive Therapy and Research, 4*(4), 325–340.

Fiszdon, J. M., Richardson, R., Greig, T., & Bell, M. D. (2007). A comparison of basic and social cognition between schizophrenia and schizoaffective disorder. *Schizophrenia Research, 91*, 117–121.

Fowles, D. C. (1988). Psychophysiology and psychopathology: A motivational approach. *Psychophysiology, 25*, 373–391.

Freud, S. (1895/1964). Studies on hysteria. In J. Strachey (Ed.), *The standard edition of the complete psychological works of Sigmund Freud* (Vol. 2). Hogarth Press.

Freud, S. (1949). Repression. In *Collected Papers* (Vol. IV). The Hogarth Press. (Original work published 1915)

Ginsburg, G. S., La Greca, A. M., & Silverman, W. K. (1998). Social anxiety in children with anxiety disorders: Relation with social and emotional functioning. *Journal of Abnormal Child Psychology, 26*, 175–185.

Gray, J. A. (1987). Perspectives on anxiety and impulsivity: A commentary. *Journal of Research in Personality, 21*, 493–509.

Gross, R. G., & Grossman, M. (2010). Executive resources. *Continuum, 16*(4), 140–152.

Hartley, C., & Phelps, E. (2010). Changing fear: The neurocircuitry of emotion regulation. *Neuropsychopharmacology, 35*, 136–146.

Isomaa, R., Vaananen, J. M., Frojd, S., Kaltiala-Heino, R., & Marttunen, M. (2013). How low is low? Low self-esteem as an indicator of internalizing psychopathology in adolescence. *Heath Education & Behavior, 40*(4), 392–399.

Jessor, R., Turbin, M. S., & Costa, F. M. (1998). Risk and protection in successful outcomes among disadvantaged adolescents. *Applied Developmental Science, 2*, 194–208.

Jones, S., & Heaven, P. (1998). Psychosocial correlates of adolescent drug-taking behavior. *Journal of Adolescence, 21*, 127–134.

Kingdon, D., & Turkington, D. (1994). *Cognitive-behavioural therapy of schizophrenia*. Lawrence A. Earlbaum Associates.

Landa, Y., Silverstein, S., Schwartz, F., & Savitz, A. (2006). Group cognitive behavioral therapy for delusions: Helping patients improve reality testing. *Journal of Contemporary Psychotherapy, 36*(1), 9–17.

Larson, C., Schaefer, H., Siegle, G., Jackson, C., Anderle, M., & Davidson, R. (2006). Fear is fast in phobic individuals; Amygdala activation in response to fear-relevant stimuli. *Biological Psychiatry, 60*(4), 410–417.

Mahurin, R. K., Velligan, D. I., & Miller, A. L. (1998). Executive-frontal lobe cognitive dysfunction in schizophrenia: A symptom subtype analysis. *Psychiatry Research, 79*, 139–149.

Mann, M., Hosman, C. M., Schaalma, H. P., & De Vries, N. K. (2004). Self-esteem in a broad-spectrum approach for mental health promotion. *Health Education & Research, 19*(4), 357–372.

Marmar, C. R., Weiss, D. S., Schlenger, W. E., Fairbank, J. A., Jordan, J. A., Kulka, R. A., & Hough, R. L. (1994). Peritraumatic dissociation and posttraumatic stress in male Vietnam theater veterans. *American Journal of Psychiatry, 151*, 902–907.

Owen, M. J. (2012). Intellectual disability and major psychiatric disorders: A continuum of neurodevelopmental causality. *British Journal of Psychiatry*, *200*(4), 268–269.

Pontzer, H. (2017). The crown joules: Energetics, ecology, and evolution in humans and other primates. *Evolutionary Anthropology*, *26*(1), 12–24.

Power, J. D., & Schlaggar, B. L. (2016). Neural plasticity across the lifespan. *Wiley Interdisciplinary Reviews Developmental Biology*, *6*(1), https://doi.org/10.1002/wdev.216

Purper-Ouakil, D., & Franc, N. (2011). Emotional dysfunction in attention deficit hyperactivity disorder. *Archives De Pediatrie*, *18*(6), 679–685.

Putman, F. W. (1985). Dissociation as an extreme response to trauma. In R. P. Kluft (Ed.), *Childhood antecedents of multiple personality* (pp. 66–97). American Psychiatric Press.

Raichlen, D. A., & Alexander, G. E. (2017). Adaptive capacity: An evolutionary neuroscience model linking exercise, cognition, and brain health. *Trends in Neuroscience*, *40*(7), 408–421.

Rapp, A. M., Langohr, K., Mutschler, D. E., & Wild, B. (2014). Irony and proverb comprehension in schizophrenia: Do female patients "dislike" ironic remarks? *Schizophrenia Research & Treatment*, *84*, 10–18.

Rouse, K. A. (1998). Longitudinal health endangering behavior among resilient and nonresilient early adolescents. *Journal of Adolescent Health*, *23*, 297–302.

Stickley, A., & Koyanagi, A. (2016). Loneliness, common mental disorders and suicidal behavior: Findings from a general population survey. *Journal of Affective Disorders*, *197*, 81–87.

Trijsburg, R., Van Spiijker, A., Van, H. L., Hesselink, A. J., & Duivenvoorden, H. J. (2000). Measuring overall defensive functioning with the defense style questionnaire. *The Journal of Nervous and Mental Disease*, *188*(7), 432–439.

Trzesniewski, K., Donnellan, B., Moffat, T., Robbins, R., Poulton, R., & Caspi, A. (2006). Low self-esteem during adolescence predicts poor health, criminal behavior, and limited economic prospects during adulthood. *Developmental Psychology*, *42*, 381–390.

Vaillant, G. (1977). *Adaptation to life*. Little, Brown and Company.

Vaillant, G. (1994). Ego mechanisms of defense and personality psychopathology. *Journal of Abnormal Psychology*, *103*(1), 44–50.

Waltereit, R., Banaschewski, T., Meyer-Lindenberg, A., & Poustka, L. (2014). Interaction of neurodevelopmental pathways and synaptic plasticity in mental retardation, autistic spectrum disorder and schizophrenia: Implication for psychiatry. *World Journal of Biological Psychiatry*, *15*(7), 507–516.

Watkins, J. G., & Watkins, H. H. (1997). *Ego states: Theory and therapy*. W. W. Norton.

Chapter 8

TRANSFERENCE

The notion of transference began with Sigmund Freud and psychoanalysis, referring to unconscious redirection of feelings toward parents to the therapist, representing a projection (Freud, 1915). According to Freud, unconscious raw material including wishes, urges, and conflicts, are transformed into conscious experience (Freud, 1915; Reed, 1990; Robbins, 2008). A transference transforms feelings and thoughts about parents into conscious experience in the present. Freud initially viewed transference as only a resistance, but realized that analysis of the transference was actually what needed to be focused on (Etchegoyen, 2005). Currently and consistent with a social cognitive perspective, transference is viewed as a normal process occurring when a person encounters someone who reminds them of an individual from their past (Andersen & Przybylinski, 2012). Hence, it really consists of transferring feelings and thoughts derived from a past social experience to a current relationship, and not just to a therapist. Based on this more general understanding, it is clear that we all have had such experiences. Perhaps a person reminds you of a past romantic partner who evokes pleasing thoughts and feelings, and those reactions are transferred onto the new person. Likewise, someone might remind you of a person you could not stand, and the negative feelings are transferred onto that individual. Transference can then be positive or negative depending on the feelings, thoughts, and images you have of the person from your past. As these examples also indicate, the experiences linked to the person from the past are typically quite strong for a transference to occur.

Regarding psychotherapy, transference is a powerful force given the intensity of feelings and thoughts about past individuals. Impediments to psychotherapy transpire due to either transference blocking progress with the client's mental health issue/s or resistance and noncompliance (mentioned in the chapter of that name), or conceivably both. Regarding the former, reactions to individuals in the client's current time frame derived from past relationships can worsen mental illness or impede recovery. For instance, a new coworker reminds the client of an abuser evoking feelings related to the abuse. Negative transference directed to the therapist, on the other hand, often represents resistance and noncompliance. Before considering each of these manifestations with examples,

DOI: 10.4324/b23346-9

we will take a look at what the literature indicates about the role of transference in psychotherapy, with a focus on transference interpretations and the impact on outcomes.

ROLE OF TRANSFERENCE IN PSYCHOTHERAPY OUTCOMES

Transference interpretation, referring to how the therapist interprets the transference and then presents this understanding to the client, plus how the client reacts, is all important. The notion being that interpreting the transference accurately and conveying this knowledge to the client, provides an opportunity to improve both relationships outside of therapy and symptoms. Reviewing transference research, almost entirely related to psychodynamic type therapies, Hoglend (2014) found that more than 30 studies reported significant associations between transference work and outcome, indicating that these interventions are active ingredients of therapy. Comparing transference work to alternative treatments, randomized controlled trials suggest that both work equally well for symptom improvement, but transference work is more effective for improving relationships and personality functioning (Hoglend, 2014). Studying personality disorder clients in long-term psychotherapy, Hoglend et al. (2011) randomly assigned 46 participants to one year of dynamic therapy with or without transference interpretations. The clients in the transference interpretation group improved significantly more in terms of core psychopathology and interpersonal functioning, with the dropout rate reduced to zero and use of health services cut by 50% (Hoglend et al., 2011). A less positive outcome came from a study by Hersoug et al. (2014), consisting of 100 clients with various mental health issues, randomly assigned to one year of psychodynamic therapy with or without transference interpretations. Outcomes in the transference group were not superior, although the researchers found that the outcome was more positive in this group for personality disorder clients in regard to specific effects (Hersoug et al., 2014). Hoglend et al. (2006) also randomly assigning 100 clients with depression, anxiety, and personality problems to dynamic therapy with or without transference interpretations, found that on several outcome variables the groups did not differ, this result countering the very positive findings from the Hoglend et al. (2011) study.

Based on the outcome research for transference interpretations, it is not simply the application that influences the effectiveness of psychotherapy, as some research shows positive outcomes compared to no transference interpretations, and other studies reveal no difference. A key factor appears to be the frequency of transference interpretations. From his review of more than 30 studies, Hoglend (2014) found that naturalistic studies show how too high a frequency of transference interpretations can have negative effects on psychotherapy outcomes. Investigating 64 patients receiving approximately 20 sessions of psychotherapy, Piper et al. (1991) discovered an inverse relationship between the proportion of transference interpretations and therapy outcomes, as well as the therapeutic alliance.

A major reason for the number of transference interpretations being related to therapy outcome, is that too frequent transference interpretations likely reduce accuracy, and incorrect interpretations can evoke negative client reactions (Connolly et al., 1999; Critis-Christoph et al., 1988; Crowder, 1972; Silberschatz et al., 1986). Supporting this proposition, Critis-Christoph et al. (1988) assessed the accuracy of 43 therapists' transference interpretations from 2 early sessions of dynamic psychotherapy. The results indicated that accuracy about main wishes and responses from others expressed in the relationship theme was related to outcome of therapy, even after controlling for the effects of general errors in treatment technique and the quality of the helping alliance (Critis-Christoph et al., 1988). The researchers noted the negative effects of high proportions of transference interpretations (Critis-Christoph et al., 1988). Studying 29 clients treated with supportive-expressive psychotherapy, Connolly et al. (1999) ascertained that high levels of transference interpretations were significantly associated with poor treatment outcome for participants with poor interpersonal functioning. Crowder (1972) performed ratings on 25 videotaped cases discovering that successful outcomes, based on pre-therapy to post-therapy changes, were characterized by less frequent transference interpretations. Concentrating on short-term dynamic psychotherapy, Schaeffer (1998) in a review of the relevant literature found that infrequent, careful, and cautious use of transference interpretations, crafting them to meet specific client characteristics and presenting problems, is effective. Identified mechanisms for this benefit consist of alliance building between the therapist and client, perseverance in therapy, and goal attainment (Schaeffer, 1998). Too frequent transference interpretations almost certainly reduce the accuracy and hence quality. In most areas of life, including psychotherapy, quality counts more than quantity, and this applies well to transference interpretations.

Various additional factors might be associated with the success or failure of transference interpretations on psychotherapy outcomes. Reviewing empirical research on transference interpretations spanning 1970–2011, Brumberg and Gumz (2012) ascertained that the results for the effectiveness are mixed and often contradictory. However, three influences emerged as most potent: amount and quality of transference interpretations, the quality of the client's interpersonal relationships (quality of object relations), and the client's immediate reaction (Brumberg & Gumz, 2012). Regarding interpersonal relationship capacity (quality of object relations), it seems that transference interpretation can be more or less effective with low or high relationship functioning. In the 2014 review, Hoglend found that transference interpretations were most effective when the client had greater difficulty with interpersonal relationships or substantial personality disorder pathology, these two scenarios often occurring together. The study by Hersoug et al. (2014) supports this perspective, as clients with low quality of object relationships and/or personality disorder showed specific positive effects of transference work. However, the Connolly et al. (1999) study discovered that high levels of transference interpretations were associated with reduced treatment outcome for clients with poor interpersonal functioning.

The focus so far has been on the therapist's performance pertaining to transference interpretations, but the client's reaction is also crucial, because when the transference interpretation resonates with the person (a palpable experience for both the client and therapist) real progress usually follows, but if the fit is not there no change or a negative reaction transpires (Brumberg & Gumz, 2012; Schaeffer, 1998). Perhaps this is one of the reasons for why interpersonal functioning (quality of object relationships) has variable effects on the success of transference interpretations: clients with poor interpersonal functioning are often very defensive rejecting interpretations, but if less defensive the interpretation can have a solid positive impact.

Most of the research reviewed has focused on psychodynamic therapies, but consistent with the social psychological perspective that transference is a normal process in relationships (Andersen & Przybylinski, 2012), it also occurs in other forms of therapy. Gelso and Bhatia (2012) indicate that transference occurs in nonanalytic psychotherapies and influences outcomes, but research is needed to better identify the process in these other therapies. Nonanalytic therapies often do not recognize, appreciate, or emphasize transference, resulting in therapists missing an opportunity to improve the therapeutic relationship and the client's progress with their mental health concerns. We will now look at transference as blocking progress with mental health issues and then as a source of resistance and noncompliance.

BLOCKING PROGRESS WITH MENTAL HEALTH ISSUES

Transference that elicits negative emotions can impede progress when it comes to virtually any mental health concern, because the condition is intensified. Depression, anxiety, trauma effects, and psychosis can all escalate limiting psychotherapy outcomes, unless effectively managed. This process is best illustrated with examples. Sue was in her early 30s when first referred to me by her family doctor, who reported that she was struggling to manage Sue's depression and anxiety, despite trying a few antidepressants and talk therapy. Sue's symptoms remained severe and she was still on disability from her work as a legal secretary. My assessment revealed a history of abuse: her father was very authoritarian and cruel laying down rules that had to be followed, and if not harsh corporal punishment was the outcome. Her mother was passive and fearful not interfering to avoid her husband's wrath, and he always justified the abuse based on perceived transgressions by Sue. Understandably, Sue left home as soon as possible around 15 years of age, and had nothing to do with her father and very little communication with her mother. She suffered from the abuse in terms of depression and anxiety, requiring medication and short-term counseling, but did not deal with the trauma issues directly. Demonstrating resilience and adaptability, she took a program for legal secretary and established a solid career. Romances were a struggle given fear and trust issues, but after initially repeating history with somewhat controlling and abusive men, she learned to avoid them and only date men who did not demonstrate such behavior. Real relationship commitment remained a problem. Sue effectively compartmentalized the abuse, a milder and adaptive form of dissociation (Bowins, 2010). Why the setback in her early 30s given the solid progress?

The assessment revealed a very powerful transference pertaining to a new lawyer at the firm. This man was a very aggressive litigation lawyer who demonstrated authoritarian behavior toward junior staff. Noting the possible transference, I suggested to her that this lawyer triggered feelings about her father that she had locked away. Sue's reaction confirmed that the transference interpretation was dead on, as she appeared shocked and then started to cry saying "Yes, he is an ass like my father!" The negative feelings toward her father that were compartmentalized had suddenly been released, and with the fear and sadness she could not perform in the presence of this lawyer, resulting in him scolding her, triggering more negative feelings, lower performance, until one day she broke down in tears at work and had to leave. The antidepressants prescribed by her family doctor could not overcome the slew of negative feelings released by this transference experience. The treatment I provided was mostly insight oriented psychotherapy working with the transference interpretation and prior abuse issues. Her feelings of weakness, shame, and sadness related to her father's abuse were gradually replaced by a sense of empowerment, aided by the fact that she had progressed with her life in terms of a solid career. She realized that she did not have to put up with the abuse, and consistent with this progression her return to work involved expressing to human resources personnel that this new lawyer does not treat staff well, and insisting on a placement with another lawyer. Expressing her concerns and being accommodated empowered her further, and she eventually was able to politely talk to this lawyer and express how she perceived his treatment of her. An added benefit was that she improved in her capacity to commit emotionally in romance, given the power she felt to control the process. Sue's mental health issues derived from early life abuse by her father were greatly intensified by the transference experience, and working with the transference interpretation enabled her to progress beyond the prior compartmentalization of the trauma.

Pam provides another example of a work based transference. My assessment revealed a pattern of perfectionism and self-criticisms, clearly derived from her parents who liked the household in order and critiqued her for being untidy and disorganized. As is common with maladaptive repetitive patterns of behavior (see the Resistance and Noncompliance chapter) she internalized this pattern and repeated it. Demonstrating a capacity to balance perfectionism with time demands, Pam functioned quite well at her accounting job, aided by a high level of conscientiousness. However, self-criticisms still followed mistakes. The problem greatly intensified when a new manager took over who turned out to be a micromanager, very critical of even the slightest mistake. In response to this management style, Pam's self-criticisms ramped up massively amplifying the impact of critiques by her manager, triggering anxiety and eventually depression.

My involvement with Pam began at this point. She was aware of how the new manager triggered the same insecure feelings her parents did—the transference. This repetition then intensified her own self-criticisms activating self-doubts and generating feelings of insecurity. We worked on the transference interpretation, and how the new manager was triggering self-doubts experienced during her childhood, based on her parents' ongoing criticisms. Realizing that she had actually internalized the pattern that hurt her, motivated efforts to establish more self-compassionate behavior with therapy providing a model of such behavior. Despite her conscientious approach to life she embraced the notion that we are all imperfect, and maybe "imperfectly perfect" in that it is mistakes that afford an opportunity to really learn and grow. This insight helped her relinquish the intense self-criticisms and be self-accepting. As is often the case with successful transference interpretations, the benefits were far-reaching. Pam realized that she had curtailed her involvements to those she could excel at to avoid her own self-criticisms, thereby limiting her life. Now being okay with mistakes and learning from them instead of beating herself up, she tried new things such as learning to play the piano. She also decided that working with a micromanager would not play out well given the transference issue plus her general competence, and she acquired a job at another accounting firm making sure to question the prospective manager about her management style before accepting the job. Almost needless to add, Pam's anxiety and depression rapidly receded.

Sue and Pam experienced a reactivation and worsening of symptoms due to transference experienced with bosses. These examples demonstrate fairly complex transference behaviors, but more circumscribed ones can also occur. For example, clients with abuse issues have experienced a reactivation of symptoms due to perceptual stimuli reminding them of the abuser. In this regard smell is powerful, such as the cologne that the abuser wore, now smelt on a store clerk, triggering feelings about the abuser. I have also seen these transference reactions based on voice, clothing, hair, body build, and other assorted features. The client reacts to the person, who is often a stranger, with feelings experienced during the abuse. Interestingly, in some instances the client reports "forgetting" about this aspect of the trauma, demonstrating how traumatic experiences are dissociated (Bowins, 2010).

The examples provided by Sue and Pam demonstrate how transference can intensify mental health problems, and effective transference interpretations are required for progress with the mental health issue/s. These examples also show how transference is not just to the therapist and can be equally powerful in response to people in the client's day to day life, with effective transference interpretations crucial for managing relationships outside of therapy.

RESISTANCE AND NONCOMPLIANCE

Transference can impede progress with psychotherapy when it produces resistance and noncompliance. In this instance, negative transference is directed toward the therapist derived from a past relationship in the client's life. The therapist will usually sense anger or resentment early on in therapy, and perhaps try and address the emotion with or without a transference interpretation. Success in addressing the emotion can be enhanced when there is an accurate transference interpretation, but not always. Steven provides an example of a "difficult" client: in the medical practice world, these individuals are referred to as "difficult patients." In his late 30s, Steven had a long history of avoidance qualifying as Avoidant Personality Disorder. Despite being healthy and quite strong he had a very sketchy record of work, usually consisting of starting a low-level job, becoming angry at a boss, having words, and being fired or quitting. He burnt out friends and most family members asking for money, and when I assessed him he had managed to acquire Ontario government support payments. From the start I sensed anger, and given that the assessment revealed parents who were critical of him since childhood and not supportive, I addressed his anger with a transference interpretation. My initial input consisted of, "I get the sense that you are angry?" His response was, "People piss me off, always wanting me to do something they want." My response was, "Is that what happens at work?" He agreed that this transpired, and I added, "We are all influenced by our caregivers and maybe your reactions to people at work are based on your parents not being supportive of what you want. Do you feel that I will act in the same way?" He listened but his emotional reaction indicated that it did not resonate. He responded, "People can just be jerks." We then discussed how based on seeing others, including me, like his parents, he might miss that people are really trying to help him progress.

Sessions following this one focused on his avoidance behavior (see the Personality Disorders chapter), helping him identify goals and foci that were not objectively threatening and offered the potential for reward. He really liked money and the things it helps acquire, and given the limited funds from the government a job involving minimal contact with people, such as landscaping, could be a huge asset. We looked at how his self-worth might be enhanced, and how it is best not to conclude that people are against him, and instead do want to see him succeed. Unfortunately, resistance emerged very fast with him missing a session and then showing up progressively later. I addressed the need to attend and reasonably on time which provoked anger, particularly when I mentioned that if he arrives too late to have a session I will have to charge for a miss. Applying the transference interpretation that he views me as an authority figure telling him what to do, did not resonate well, nor did going over how we all have to live with boundaries. One time he arrived so close to the end of the session that I told him that as mentioned he will have to pay. His response was that I am a "f…ing jerk," and he left the office slamming the door. I cannot say that I was sorry to see him go, a reaction I am certain most people in his life feel.

Transferences can be somewhat more complicated, unlike with Steven, having both positive and negative aspects. In his early 40s when first assessed, Manuel provides an example of a more complex transference. He had a neurological condition from childhood that impaired his movements and speech. Lacking confidence in himself he never tried to advance and only had odd jobs that were not challenging. During the assessment, he identified this as a major concern and expressed that he knew he could do more, and would appreciate the boost to his self-worth. Aware of programs that hire people with disabilities, some offering solid opportunities, I suggested that he might consider this option and I would fill out forms supporting the application. He liked the idea, but it was clear that he was dragging his heels so to speak in following up on it. During one session, I noted him smiling at me in quite a pronounced fashion. Addressing it as something potentially significant, I asked him to share his thoughts. His response indicated a positive transference: "You remind me of my father who has always believed that I can do more and encourages me. That's why I wanted to continue with you." Pleased but sensing a "but" I asked, "Why are you hesitating to apply to that program then?" A more negative transference emerged at this point: "I just feel that I cannot do what my father and you want, and do not like feeling pushed." He then expressed how he resisted taking the next steps of acquiring an application form and filling it out. Despite going over how it is his decision and trying his best will not disappoint me, nor I felt certain his father, his self-doubts proved overwhelming and he would not advance with the application. Sessions faded to infrequent supportive ones, with him maintaining a non-challenging part time job.

The focus in this chapter and book is on impediments to progress with psychotherapy, but transference reactions can also be positive, and equally powerful as negative ones, when it comes to mental health issues. Katerina provides an example of a potent positive transference. In her late 20s, Katerina experienced several mental health issues consisting of polysubstance abuse, anxiety, depression, and anger-aggression usually in the context of substance abuse. Demonstrating solid personality features including conscientiousness, extroversion, agreeableness, and limited reactivity, she maintained a technology job with good performance reviews, but no upward mobility related to self-doubts. Katerina had a very dysfunctional childhood, with a schizophrenic mother and a low functioning father who held odd religious ideas and was very cruel. As an aside, females with schizophrenia are more likely to marry than males with this illness, but often end up with quite dysfunctional partners. Katerina's parents did not get along and during a psychotic episode when her mother threatened to harm the children, they separated with her father gaining custody.

From this point, he immersed himself in fringe religions and expected the children to be adherent to the beliefs. Failure to recite religious passages accurately and other violations resulted in harsh punishment, such as no meals for that day, being locked in a closet, and the strap. Katerina ran away from home at 13 years of age and immersed herself in the drug culture. Years later she found herself in a depressive rut with routine work during the week, intense partying on the weekend, anxious and depressed feelings ongoing, combined with moments of anger and aggression when using substances.

Sensing that she was in a rut, Katerina sought a psychiatric assessment. Clinicians might assume that her primary issue was personality disorder, and in particular borderline, but this did not appear to be the case. She demonstrated mature defense mechanisms with a great and appropriate sense of humor, sublimation of negative feelings into work and music, was able to suppress negative feelings and aggressive urges in the moment, and was very helpful to others showing altruism. Consistent with the defense mechanism model of personality disorder presented in the Personality Disorders chapter, there was very little use of immature defenses, and hence Borderline Personality Disorder was not a good fit. Confirming this perspective, her friendships were reasonable, although with others who abused alcohol and various drugs, and she demonstrated a very stable work record. The notion of normal personality traits predisposing to personality disorders is relevant, as she showed low to moderate reactivity, and not the intense reactivity (neuroticism) seen with borderline problems. Conscientiousness, extroversion, and agreeableness were also protective against a formal personality disorder.

Transference emerged in therapy based on her perceiving me as the caring and attentive father she never had. With positive transference, there is no need for transference interpretations, although some therapists might disagree with this. The transference remained robust and was undoubtedly a key factor in her rapid progression, along with her positive normal personality features and medication for anxiety and depression. She gave up alcohol and party drugs while maintaining friendships with a few people she previously partied with, something that usually does not occur and likely only transpired due to her agreeable friendly nature. She shifted interests to more progressive pursuits including learning a new language and courses to upgrade her skills. Working with her self-doubts and appreciating that I believed in her abilities, she sought a promotion and eventually became a manger excelling at it given her vast experience and conscientiousness. She also faced her weight issue that initially we thought might be partly medication related, but was not given how it persisted long after the medications were withdrawn. She is still working on this problem but is prepared to do what she must for her health. The positive transference was a major factor in her incredible progress that has persisted. Katerina illustrates how positive transference can be a robust force in mental health and psychotherapy progression. A key reason for why this transpires is how positive transference and the therapeutic alliance mutually reinforce one another: a positive transference within therapy clearly strengthens the thera-peutic alliance, which in turn advances the positive transference feelings, bol-stering the therapeutic alliance, and so on and so forth, with the activation and intensification of these pro-therapy forces enhancing progress.

An interesting aspect of transference interpretations is that it typically requires a certain number of sessions to be worked on, although transference can emerge right away even during the assessment. To benefit from transfer-ence work both the client and therapist must persist for more than a session or two. In some instances, the therapist will terminate the process when sensing negativity, based on how initial negative responses by the client usually lead to a poor therapeutic alliance impairing outcomes. However, if the transference interpretation, or just addressing the negative affect, yields a positive response then a solid therapeutic alliance can grow. Some clients will just stop after the first or second session if they feel negativity, attributing it to a poor fit. If the client perseveres there is the potential for a negative transference to be worked on yielding real therapeutic gains.

WORKING WITH TRANSFERENCE

Transference can facilitate psychotherapy outcomes if positive and hinder it if negative. Impediments to psychotherapy related to transference involve either blocks to progress with mental health issues or resistance and noncompliance. In both instances the therapist and client play a role in the end result.

Therapist Role

The most crucial aspect is to be open to the concept of transference and look for signs of it. This advice will seem obvious to therapists working from a psy-chodynamic perspective, but in this day and age of short-term interventions it is often not emphasized in training, while still being just as potent. Given that transference interpretations best involve quality over quantity, if you are not sure that it is transpiring the best strategy is to, first, discuss it with a colleague, and second, present it to the client as a possibility rather than a statement of fact. I believe that it is always wise to present transference interpretations as possi-bilities, but some are so obvious, such as with Sue, that the confidence level in expressing it can be high. Be aware or even wary of presenting dubious transfer-ence interpretations to disagreeable clients with a history of anger and aggression, as the response might not be what you hoped for. Often it is best to wait until the client has progressed, but failure to progress with therapy due to resistance and noncompliance can transpire until the transference issue is resolved, creating a conundrum that can feel like a tightrope walk. This is where experience and being lenient on yourself as a therapist come in handy, as does consultation with a colleague or two. Despite your most professional approach transference inter-pretations do not always lead to therapeutic gains, even if accurate.

From the perspective of transference either blocking progress with mental health issues or resistance and noncompliance, noting the distinction can help as they entail a somewhat different therapeutic focus: the former emphasizes how the transference has worsened a mental illness (or illnesses) and addressing it provides ways to advance mental health regarding the given condition/s, while with resistance and noncompliance the focus is more on how the transference impairs working with the therapist, and from this the development of a solid therapeutic alliance. Appreciating the relevance and power of positive transference is also important, as therapy can move along very nicely when this transpires, largely because the positive transference and therapeutic alliance mutually reinforce each other, thereby activating robust forces for psychotherapy progress.

Client Role

Transference reactions are largely unconscious, and so are usually not realized consciously until the therapist makes a transference interpretation. The key here is to be open to these interpretations and resist the urge to reject them. Since you have not been aware of the transference, it might seem like a strange notion but that does not mean it is inaccurate, and working with the transference interpretation can greatly enhance progress with therapy. Conversely, rejecting and not working with transference interpretations can leave you stuck in a very deep rut, with failure to progress in terms of your mental health issue and psychotherapy. Persevering when negative feelings toward the therapist are experienced is then important, as is raising these feelings with the therapist, an action that can prompt a transference interpretation. A guide to the accuracy of these interpretations consists of your emotional reaction: if there is no real reaction the chances are reduced that it is relevant, unless you are dissociated from your feelings, but if the emotional response is strong the transference interpretation is quite likely spot on. If you do not feel that it fits, then be assertive about this belief, and if accurate work with the therapist regarding it.

SUMMARY NOTE

The notion of transference has a long and robust history in psychotherapy reflecting its relevance, although with short-term packaged interventions transference reactions are often missed and not interpreted to the detriment of the client. Initially conceived by psychoanalysts as a process only occurring in therapy, transference also transpires when the client encounters someone who reminds them of a person from their past, in line with a social cognitive perspective. The majority of research on transference focuses on psychoanalytic type therapies, despite the relevance of transference beyond this psychotherapy setting. Review studies support the perspective that it is a very active ingredient in psychotherapy capable of improving symptoms, interpersonal relationships, and personality issues. As with many things in life, quality of transference interpretations appears to be far more important than quantity, with fewer accurate interpretations yielding the best outcome. The client's reaction to the transference interpretation is crucial, as when it fits and resonates with the individual real progress is likely.

Transference can impede psychotherapy by either blocking progress with mental health issues or resistance and noncompliance, although most therapists only focus on the latter. The distinction is relevant as it provides a somewhat different therapeutic focus, the former on how the transference worsens mental illness and addressing it suggests ways to advance these concerns, while resistance and noncompliance emphasize how the transference impairs working with the therapist and hence the formation of a robust therapeutic alliance. A take home message is that transference is a potent psychotherapy force advancing outcomes if positive and hindering them if negative, and it is definitely helpful to address negative transference and ride the wave of positive transference.

REFERENCES

Andersen, S. M., & Przybylinski, E. (2012). Experiments on transference relations: Implications for treatment. *Psychotherapy (Chicago)*, 49(3), 370–383.

Bowins, B. E. (2010). Repetitive maladaptive behavior: Beyond repetition compulsion. *American Journal of Psychoanalysis*, 70, 282–298.

Brumberg, J., & Gumz, A. (2012). Transference interpretations and how they work: A systematic review. *Z Psychosomatic Medicine Psychotherapy*, 58(3), 219–235.

Connolly, M., Cris-Christoph, P., Shappell, S., Barber, J., Luborsky, L., & Shaffer, C. (1999). Relationship of transference interpretations to outcome in the early sessions of brief supportive-expressive psychotherapy. *Psychotherapy Research*. https://doi.org/10.1080/10503309912331332881

Critis-Christoph, P., Cooper, A., & Luborsky, L. (1988). The accuracy of therapists' interpretations and the outcome of dynamic psychotherapy. *Journal of Consulting and Clinical Psychology*, 56(4), 490–495.

Crowder, J. E. (1972). Relationship between therapist and client interpersonal behaviors and psychotherapy outcome. *Journal of Counseling Psychology*, 19(1), 68–75.

Etchegoyen, H. (2005). *The fundamentals of psychoanalytic technique*. Karnak Books.

Freud, S. (1915). The unconscious. *Standard Edition*, 14, 166–215.

Gelso, C. J., & Bhatia, A. (2012). Crossing theoretical lines: The role and effect of transference in nonanalytic psychotherapies. *Psychotherapy (Chicago)*, 49(3), 384–390.

Hersoug, A. G., Ulberg, R., & Hoglend, P. (2014). When is transference work useful in psychodynamic psychotherapy? Main results of the first experimental study of transference work (FEST). *Contemporary Psychoanalysis*, 50(1–2), 156–174.

Hoglend, P. (2014). Exploration of the patient-therapist relationship in psychotherapy. *American Journal of Psychotherapy*, 171(10), 1056–1066.

Hoglend, P., Amlo, S., Marble, A., Bogwald, K. P., Sorbye, O., Sjaastad, M. C., et al. (2006). Analysis of the patient-therapist relationship in dynamic psychotherapy: An experimental study of transference interpretations. *The American Journal of Psychiatry*, 163(10), 1739–1746.

Hoglend, P., Dahl, H. S., Hersoug, A. G., Lorentzen, S., & Perry, J. C. (2011). Long-term effects of transference interpretation in dynamic psychotherapy of personality disorders. *European Psychiatry*, *26*(7), 419–424.

Piper, W. E., Azim, H. F., & Joyce, A. S. (1991). Transference interpretations, therapeutic alliance, and outcome in short-term individual psychotherapy. *Archives of General Psychiatry*, *48*(10), 946–953.

Reed, G. S. (1990). The transference neurosis in Freud's writings. *Journal of the American Psychoanalytic Association*, *38*(2), 423–450.

Robbins, M. (2008). Primary mental expression: Freud, Klein, and beyond. *Journal of the American Psychoanalytic Association*, *56*(1), 177–202.

Schaeffer, J. A. (1998). Transference and countertransference interpretations: Harmful or helpful in short-term dynamic therapy? *American Journal of Psychotherapy*, *52*(1), 1–17.

Silberschatz, G., Fretter, P. B., & Curtis, J. T. (1986). How do interpretations influence the process of psychotherapy? *Journal of Consulting and Clinical Psychology*, *54*(5), 646–652.

Section II

Therapist Influences

Chapter 9

COUNTERTRANSFERENCE

Given that the therapist is a person, and hopefully not replaced by an artificial intelligence system, past relationships can influence feelings and behavior toward the client. This occurrence is known as countertransference, the therapist version of transference we covered in the Client Influences section. As with transference, the notion of countertransference arose with Sigmund Freud, who initially viewed it as an unconscious interference with an analyst's ability to understand the patient derived from unresolved issues (Abend, 1989). From this perspective, the therapist's past issues are a reactive mental state creating an obstacle to progress in psychotherapy with the potential to damage the client, such that it needs to be overcome (Bouchard et al., 1995). This earlier psychodynamic view of countertransference has shifted to include broader therapist responses to the client, and the notion that these reactions are somewhat shaped by the client, thereby providing valuable information, and not just obstacles to be overcome (Abend, 1989; Bouchard et al., 1995). Countertransference can inform regarding the client's personality and predominant behavior patterns, limit therapeutic interventions, influence client resistance and the therapeutic alliance, and impact therapy outcomes (Cartwright, 2011; Colli & Ferri, 2015; Geltner, 2006). Derived from social psychology, attribution theory is relevant as it shows how biases can lead observers to conclude that certain traits apply to others (Lewis, 2009). For instance, attractive people are usually ascribed superior traits such as integrity. Therapists often apply these common biases to clients, and also those derived from their own life, such as assuming that a client who is similar to a pleasing person they know will have good traits and intentions (Lewis, 2009).

Supporting the importance of countertransference is a study by Hayes et al. (2018) involving three meta-analyses: the first indicates that countertransference can adversely impact psychotherapy outcomes, the second that effective management attenuates negative effects, and the third that successful management is related to improved psychotherapy outcomes. In an earlier work, also applying a few meta-analyses, Hayes et al. (2011) found that countertransference is inversely and moderately related to psychotherapy outcomes (more countertransference worse outcomes), and that successfully managing

DOI: 10.4324/b23346-11

it contributes to better outcomes. Crowder (1972) assessing 25 videotaped sessions of psychotherapy, determined that successful therapists exhibited fewer countertransference responses than less successful therapists, and particularly during later sessions.

Too frequent countertransference responses do appear to impair psychotherapy outcomes. However, qualitative aspects of countertransference are also a very important consideration. Applying a systematic review of 25 mostly psychoanalytic studies distilled from 1,081, Machado et al. (2014) found that positive countertransference, referring to feelings of closeness to the patient, correlated with positive outcomes, including symptom improvement, and a good therapeutic alliance. As pertains to the management of countertransference, Gelso and Hayes (2001) identified therapist self-insight, self-integration, anxiety management, empathy, and conceptualizing ability as crucial. Evaluating these five aspects of countertransference management, Gelso et al. (2002) assessed 32 therapist trainees having their supervisors complete the Countertransference Factors Inventory, and both trainees and supervisors rate the outcome of psychotherapy. Anxiety management and conceptualizing skills were positively related to trainee and supervisor ratings of outcome, and self-integration to trainee assessment of outcome (Gelso et al., 2002). Demonstrating how complex the qualitative aspects of countertransference are, Westerling et al. (2019) evaluated 119 client-therapist relationships, finding that client attachment anxiety was associated with decreased therapist rated parental/protective and special/overinvolved countertransference throughout therapy sessions, while decreases in client attachment anxiety linked to increases in therapist reported overwhelmed/disorganized countertransference. Certain personality characteristics of clients including high avoidance, exploitable-overly nurturing, intrusive, domineering, vindictive, and cold, are related to less positive and greater negative therapist countertransference (Rossberg et al., 2008).

More research is required to distill the valid qualitative aspects of countertransference linked to psychotherapy outcomes, but it is clear that positive countertransference does improve outcomes, whereas negative countertransference that is not managed effectively impairs the success of psychotherapy. As with transference, infrequent, careful, and cautious use crafting countertransference interpretations to specific client characteristics and presenting problems is most optimal (Schaeffer, 1998). This scenario is understandable given how complex countertransference (and transference) is, with the client influencing the therapist's reaction and experiences of the therapist projected onto the client. The notion of therapist's reaction to the client has led to a common distinction between countertransference and "counter-reaction" but this is in my opinion not valid, because every therapist has emotional reactions to clients (and others in their life) consistent with emotional information processing, and hence there is nothing unique about this. However, reactions to clients based on experiences with others in the therapist's life is distinct, validating the notion of countertransference.

I will now provide some countertransference examples derived from my own practice, that demonstrate how both therapist experiences and client influences play out.

CASE EXAMPLES

A very common countertransference is based on the client's use of idealization/ devaluation, an immature defense covered in the Personality Disorders chapter. This defense often manifests in the context of Borderline Personality Disorder. Sheela, an early-30s woman, experienced a traumatic childhood with both her mother and a sibling dying of cancer. Worsening matters, her father was ill-equipped to be a supportive parent, growing up with emotionally distant caregivers and poverty. When Sheela needed emotional support the most, her father could not provide it. As she entered adolescence she discovered that teenage boys would be supportive until they were sexually satisfied, and then abandoned her, a repetition of losing her mother and sibling. Sheela demonstrated several immature psychological defenses including splitting, idealization/ devaluation, and acting out. The most prominent early in therapy was idealization without the devaluation. She was excessively complementary and quick to identify and acknowledge my positive features. Naturally, I found myself warming to her and feeling uplifted. We are a social species and positive feedback from others is rewarding.

Within the context of countertransference, Sheela reminded me of supportive people over the course of my life, and was a very welcome break from the stressful clients. Fortunately, being aware of psychological defense mechanisms and the nature of idealization with the devaluation part likely to follow, I worked with the countertransference, although admit that I went along with the idealization ride for a short while. Appreciating that the idealization derived from a wish for a caring and supportive parent, and how it was reinforced by the positive attention she received from males, we looked at her history and how much she needed support given the losses she sustained, with this need met at least briefly from sexual romances. Therapy took an interesting twist at this point: one day she walked in wearing a nicer outfit than usual (her clothing was always stylish but not seductive) exclaiming, "We need to change the relationship! You sit there" pointing to the seat she usually sat in, "and I'll sit in your seat." Curiosity won over and I went along with this suggestion. Comfortable that she had achieved this change, she then proposed that we have a different relationship as a couple, and more equal, the change in seating reflecting this. Exploring what this meant, she expressed pleasure at the attention I paid to her. Tapping into the countertransference, I indicated that I found her attention and positive comments to be pleasing as well. It is easy to envision at this juncture how failing to work with countertransference (and transference) can lead to therapy disasters, whereas working with these processes can yield real psychotherapy progress. We discussed how the possibility she raised would only repeat her pattern of wishing for emotional support, seeking and briefly finding it in males, and then being disappointed when it did not work out, with anger and negativity following. Being quite psychologically minded, she listened and acknowledged that a pattern of intense romance followed by let-downs and withdrawal characterized her life. I suggested that the therapy rela-tionship might be a better alternative, enabling me to provide support and help her change the pattern that has not been effective. To her benefit, she engaged and progressed very well in therapy, and without the devaluation of my role that would have been inevitable if a failed alternative relationship transpired.

It has been commented that creating a safe therapeutic space allowing for creative exploration of past and present is crucial, and also how the therapist must tolerate some ambiguity (Adler, 1994). If I refused to go along with the chair change during that session, Sheela would likely have felt opposed and ineffectual, leading to anger and devaluation. Instead, a safe therapeutic space for creative exploration was provided yielding powerful countertransference and transference interpretations, proving pivotal to the progress of therapy. It has also been proposed that therapy for borderline personality disorder ben-efits from countertransference work, and that the therapist's recognition and capacity to deal with these issues is crucial to treatment progress (Meissner, 1982–1983).

Projective identification comprises another immature psychological defense mechanism that is relevant for countertransference reactions, even capa-ble of drawing the therapist into various forms of acting out (Waska, 1999). Borderline Personality Disorder is a context where projective identification is common, although frequently unrecognized to the detriment of therapy and the therapist's mental wellbeing. With projective identification, the client pro-jects negative states that are hard to identify with onto the therapist, as well as others in their life, and once the person acts in the projected fashion the client is able to identify with the negative state and hence settles emotionally. A common negative state is anger. Daniella, a mid-20s woman with Borderline Personality Disorder, provides an example of a client who frequently utilized this defense without any conscious awareness. The trauma she experienced in childhood consisted of having to move away from her parents, and live with grandparents when the communist system fell in Eastern Europe. Her parents struggled to find consistent work and could not afford help, hence Daniella and her siblings had to live quite far away in another part of the country for a few years. These new caregivers were not objectively abusive, but engaged in strict discipline without much emotional support. Daniella experienced the shift in living arrangement as abandonment by her parents, and losing emotional sup-port given the cold nature of her grandparents.

Usually quite pleasant and engaging, Daniella experienced anger when faced with any hint of abandonment, perceiving it as damaging and violat-ing due to her background. However, anger was not in her presentation, and instead she calmly made highly irritating and abrasive comments, such as

"You don't really seem to care about your patients." She also utilized idealization/devaluation, and to some extent these comments were devaluations, but the unemotional expression suggested that more was going on. Possessing solid intelligence and social skills, Daniella was very creative in these comments and I found myself getting angry, thinking about annoying people encountered in my life including clients. It was only when I expressed some anger in my tone, derived from both her behavior and my own past annoying relationships, that the comments stopped and she appeared to settle in terms of less muscle tension, which she noted. We looked at how anger was impossible to express during childhood, given that her grandparents were stern and not emotionally supportive. Expressions of anger were punished blocking their expression. We examined how she very creatively and unconsciously for the most part, finds ways to elicit anger in me and others.

Projective identification is a complex psychological defense and it can be challenging to work with, but Daniella grasped the concept. I went over how she can express anger, but not formal aggression, in therapy sessions safely without punishment, and how I would much prefer this to the negative emotion buildup. Her verbal skills assisted in expressing anger in an emotional and assertive fashion, affording the opportunity to explore the damage and violation theme, and how it related to her early life subjective trauma. Progress with this shift from projective identification to assertive expression of negative emotions had far reaching positive consequences, as she found that people no longer abandoned her, and she came to understand why her history of abandonment repeated largely through projective identification. Of significance, of all the immature defenses, projective identification can be one of the most annoying and challenging to work with as it is difficult to catch, explain, and shift, but when this is successful a major impediment to psychotherapy progress is removed. Interpretation is central to shifting projective identification to a mutual understanding (Waska, 1999), and this of course is dependent on the therapist recognizing what is transpiring.

Countertransference can tap into numerous aspects of a therapist's life, and one that is highly relevant to the nature of psychotherapy is money. Psychotherapy is a business, unless you happen to be independently wealthy and money is not a concern, and financial aspects do trigger feelings. One therapist known to me allowed a client to defer payments for several sessions, but with the understanding that payment would follow with a new job. When the client dropped out of therapy and refused to pay, the therapist had a collection agency seek the money. This less than ideal action resulted in a formal complaint launched by the client to the therapist's governing body, and a reprimand from this organization. The therapist was sensitive to not being paid, the negative feelings amplified by past violations of this nature, leading to poor judgment and adverse consequences. Appreciating the relevance of money issues in therapy, Shapiro and Ginzberg (2006) recommend a thorough self-examination, including an ethical framework for decision making about money matters, to safeguard against problems resulting from therapist's and client's unconscious relationship to money. It is also suggested that clear policies are in place pertaining to money matters in therapy, such as setting and paying of fees, third party payments, and the handling of payments (Shapiro & Ginzberg, 2006).

My own version of money matters takes the form of charging for non-insured services. In the Ontario health care system psychotherapy sessions by medical doctor therapists are covered by government payments. However, several extra services must be charged for outside of the system, such as filling out forms. I did not bother charging for any of these services until several years of cutbacks from the government and rising costs of running my practice, shifted the balance. Of note, I do not charge these fees to clients who are strictly on government support. In keeping with the recommendations by Shapiro and Ginzberg (2006), I explain the nature of these payments during the assessment and have them sign and date the agreement. One client, Tom, provoked quite a strong countertransference reaction. In his early-40s with a very well paying and completely stable government job, Tom was not at all hard up for money as the saying goes. However, he expressed an unwillingness to pay for these uninsured service fees. During early sessions, it emerged that Tom was worried about many unrealistic scenarios including financial hardship. We went over how people perceive things that are not in keeping with reality, and given his financial circumstances placing him in the upper 80% of the population, this fear is not realistic. He listened but also expressed painful cheapness in his dealing with other people and stores. Very negative feelings that can best be described as contempt, derived from a mixture of anger and disgust, arose within me. Another earlier client experience seemingly popped out, this involving a mid-30s man who had the fortune of his father handing him a lucrative chain of stores cost free! One time he missed a session and I indicated that as per agreement he will have to cover the fee, as I cannot bill the government system for missed sessions. He refused stating that the miss was an emergency, that when prompted he cited as his wife's mother having a rapidly scheduled appointment with a prospective nursing home. I indicated that this absolutely does not qualify as an emergency, the signed agreement specifying a life-threatening or severe medical problem, and he will have to pay. He refused and we ended sessions. Even writing this I still feel contempt at the injustice and lack of morality, considering that this person was a multimillionaire and would not cover one missed session. One can only imagine how he would treat employees. Getting back to Tom, I worked with my countertransference feelings by understanding his perspective, that despite there not being any objective evidence, he felt insecure financially and in regard to other matters. Instead of a therapy rupture, we worked on altering his excessive threat and danger perceptions fostering progress in therapy.

A more positive tone example of countertransference involves a late-20s man, Byron, who presented with depression and self-criticisms related to career and lack of progress in life. He had completed both undergraduate and Master's degrees in linguistics, but found himself only able to secure a minimum wage job, not an uncommon scenario for young people these days. He described his father and mother as quite critical, insisting that he had to do at least one university degree. During high school, he indicated to them that he would prefer to go to a community college to study film, which was an interest if not a passion. Unfortunately, they did not see this as worthwhile and he felt too guilty to resist and move in the direction that felt right, instead entering into university. With no career prospects after the undergraduate degree, he did the Master's degree, although not really interested, discovering once again that it did not lead to a good job. The dysfunctional pattern of criticisms demonstrated by his parents had been internalized, and he continually put himself down for the lack of career success and weakness for not following his own path. When I started to work with him I was somewhat concerned about the education and career motivation of my children, and warmed up to this young man given his motivation and concerns about his own success. My stance was supportive indicating that adaptability is key to success in life and mental health. With his interest in film and the robust film industry in Toronto, his career preference was an ideal option, and not at all too late given that many people retrain in their 30s and 40s. We also went over the importance of self-acceptance (see the Impaired States and Processes for Mental Health chapter for Adaptability and Self-Acceptance). He could see how he was using a sledge hammer of sorts against the foundation of his own being via the self-criticisms. The technique of self-esteem journaling was applied to help bolster his self-esteem, self-concept, and hence self-acceptance. A positive transference transpired with him seeing me as a parent supportive of his career ambitions, assisting in him internalizing my supportive input and pattern. He then embarked on retraining for the film industry. His depression gradually cleared accompanied by increasing self-acceptance.

My choice of countertransference examples covers a variety of client issues and scenarios routinely encountered by therapists, including positive and negative reactions to clients, all relating to past relationships in my life. The examples demonstrate the information value of countertransference, both pertaining to the client and therapist. To optimize countertransference management there are some strategies that therapists can adopt, and with practice become better at.

WORKING WITH COUNTERTRANSFERENCE

For the therapist to work with countertransference, conscious awareness is a prerequisite. If a therapist is not aware of their own reactions to clients, then it will be impossible to derive any information and direction from this powerful psychotherapy influence. Awareness requires that the therapist focus not only on the client but on themselves, and making the challenge even more complicated, pay attention to the interaction, a topic that will be discussed further in the Interactive Influences section. With more experience providing psychotherapy and engaging this divided attention, countertransference work can help remove obstacles to progress and assist with self-discovery. I have noted based on my own experience and that of other psychotherapists who have continued to practice over several years, that self-discovery, or almost self-psychotherapy, follows from providing therapy for clients, and countertransference interpretations contribute significantly to this occurrence. Rosenblatt (2009) indicates that providing psychotherapy can be therapeutic to the therapist even when not intentionally sought, based on how therapists expose aspects of themselves that are accepted by clients when healing occurs, providing the therapist with a new sense of their own life.

With conscious awareness applied to your own responses to the client, openness and acceptance are the next strategies. Therapists are people like clients and will invariably have emotional reactions, and also responses linked to prior relationship experiences. Being open to this inevitable scenario and accepting it fosters progress in psychotherapy, whereas being closed and non-accepting can impede progress sometimes with disastrous results. For example, erotic countertransference feelings toward certain clients provide important information regarding the client, and also personal vulnerabilities. If ignored, then boundaries can and not uncommonly are crossed damaging the client and scuttling the therapist's career. Instead, by working with this information progress in therapy transpires, and also self-acceptance for the therapist. Indeed, powerful countertransference feelings of any nature typically reveal key information about the client and therapist.

Applying the information obtained from countertransference (and transference) is the next step. One debatable issue is whether or not to raise countertransference feelings with the client? The answer might depend on the preference and particular experience of the therapist, and nature of the given client. Personally, I do not find that it is necessary to share countertransference and it can overwhelm clients. More important is applying this information to guide the direction of therapy. In general terms, appreciate that countertransference arises in response to behavior and features of clients, and hence provides important information about them. Specifically, there are numerous options some covered in the client examples. Immature defense mechanism usage can be addressed and mature defense mechanisms fostered, as with Sheela (idealization/devaluation) and Daniella (projective identification). Money issues are relevant to almost all psychotherapists and can provoke countertransference reactions based on experiences with prior clients as with Tom, and using the information can assist in helping the client deal with issues such as anxiety and worry. Positive countertransference responses as with Byron can feel like riding a nice wave, an analogy that anyone who has surfed can appreciate, and applied strategically the intervention provides a rewarding experience for both the client and therapist. Erotic type countertransference reactions are very important to work with, as if ignored and acted on psychotherapy disasters ensue, but if applied to the client, attachment and other relationship issues can be remedied. Of note, some therapists feel guilt or other negative emotional reactions to certain countertransference feelings, but within the context of self-acceptance and its important role in mental health, appreciate that these feelings are inevitable and instead of self-criticisms, work with the information to the benefit of the client's and your own mental health!

SUMMARY NOTE

The notion of countertransference arose with Sigmund Freud, who initially viewed it as an unconscious interference with an analyst's ability to understand the patient derived from unresolved issues. This earlier psychodynamic view of countertransference has shifted to include broader therapist responses to the client, and the notion that these reactions are somewhat shaped by the client, thereby providing valuable information. Countertransference can inform regarding the client's personality and predominant behavior patterns, limit therapeutic interventions, influence client resistance and the therapeutic alliance, and impact therapy outcomes. Positive countertransference improves outcomes, whereas negative countertransference that is not managed effectively impairs the success of psychotherapy. As with transference, infrequent, careful, and cautious use crafting countertransference interpretations to specific client characteristics and presenting problems is most optimal. Working with transference entails conscious awareness, openness and acceptance, and applying the information in a strategic fashion as in the case examples provided.

REFERENCES

Abend, S. M. (1989). Countertransference and psychoanalytic technique. *Psychoanalytic Quarterly*, *58*(3), 374–395.

Adler, G. (1994). Transference, countertransference, and abuse in psychotherapy. *Harvard Review of Psychiatry*, *2*(3), 151–159.

Bouchard, M. A., Normandin, L., & Sequin, M. H. (1995). Countertransference as instrument and obstacle: A comprehensive and descriptive framework. *Psychoanalytic Quarterly*, *64*(4), 717–745.

Cartwright, C. (2011). Transference, countertransference, and reflective practice in cognitive therapy. *Clinical Psychologist*. https://doi: 10.1111/j.1742-9552.2011.00030.x

Colli, A., & Ferri, M. (2015). Patient personality and therapist countertransference. *Current Opinion in Psychiatry*, *28*(1), 46–56.

Crowder, J. E. (1972). Relationship between therapist and client interpersonal behaviors and psychotherapy outcome. *Journal of Counseling Psychology*, *19*(1), 68–75.

Gelso, C. J., & Hayes, J. A. (2001). Countertransference management. *Psychotherapy: Theory, Research, Practice, Training*, *38*(4), 418–422.

Gelso, C. J., Latts, M. G., Gomez, M. J., & Fassinger, R. E. (2002). Countertransference management and therapy outcome: An initial evaluation. *Journal of Clinical Psychology*. https://doi.org/10.1002/jclp.2010

Geltner, P. (2006). The concept of objective countertransference and its role in a two-person psychology. *American Journal of Psychoanalysis*, 66(1), 25–42.

Hayes, J. A., Gelso, C. J., & Goldberg, S. (2018). Countertransference management and effective psychotherapy: Meta-analytic findings. *Psychotherapy (Chic)*, 54(4), 496–507.

Hayes, J. A., Gelso, C. J., & Hummel, A. M. (2011). Managing countertransference. *Psychotherapy*, 48(1), 88–97.

Lewis, J. I. (2009). The crossroads of countertransference and attribution theory: Reinventing clinical training within an evidence-based treatment world. *American Journal of Psychoanalysis*, 69(2), 106–120.

Machado, D., Coelho, F. M., Giacomelli, A. D., Donassolo, M. A., Abitante, M. S., Dall'Agnol, T., et al. (2014). Systematic review of studies about countertransference in adult psychotherapy. *Trends in Psychiatry and Psychotherapy*. https://doi.org/10.1590/2237-6089-2014-1004

Meissner, W. W. (1982–1983). Notes on countertransference in borderline conditions. *International Journal of Psychoanalysis*, 9, 89–124.

Rosenblatt, P. C. (2009). Providing psychotherapy can be therapeutic for a therapist. *American Journal of Psychotherapy*, 63(2), 169–181.

Rossberg, J. I., Sigmund, K., Pedersen, G., & Friis, S. (2008). Specific personality traits evoke different countertransference reactions: An empirical study. *The Journal of Nervous and Mental Disease*, 196(9), 702–708.

Schaeffer, J. A. (1998). Transference and countertransference interpretations: Harmful or helpful in short-term dynamic therapy? *American Journal of Psychotherapy*, 52(1), 1–17.

Shapiro, E. L., & Ginzberg, R. (2006). Buried treasure: Money, ethics, and countertransference in group therapy. *International Journal of Group Psychotherapy*, 56(4), 477–494.

Waska, R. T. (1999). Projective identification, countertransference, and the struggle for understanding over acting out. *Journal of Psychotherapy Practice and Research*, 8(2), 155–161.

Westerling, T. W., Drinkwater, R., Laws, H., Stevens, H., Orega, S., Goodman, D., et al. (2019). Patient attachment and therapist countertransference in psychodynamic psychotherapy. *Psychoanalytic Psychology*, 36(1), 73–81.

Chapter 10

EMOTIONAL FACTORS

Given the prominence of emotions in human psychological functioning, it is understandable that emotional factors pertaining to the therapist have a major impact on the progress of psychotherapy. When emotional functioning is impaired, progress is impeded and when intact psychotherapy can progress well. Emotional capacity and stability stand out as most significant, with empathy flowing from solid capacity. We will now look at the role played by emotional capacity and stability.

EMOTIONAL CAPACITY

For an understanding of emotional capacity, we must revisit emotion information processing covered in the Expectations chapter. Primary emotions are universal in people (and in many mammals and primates) due to how they relate to core evolutionary relevant circumstances referred to as deep structures (Boucher & Carlson, 1980; Ekman, 1972):

Happiness—gain or success (Beck, 1991; Shaver et al., 1987).
Interest—detection of something offering the potential for reward (Izard, 1991).
Sadness—loss (Beck, 1991; Eley & Stevenson, 2000; Finlay-Jones & Brown, 1981).
Fear—threat or danger (Eley & Stevenson, 2000; Finlay-Jones & Brown, 1981; Shaver et al., 1987).
Anger—violation or damage (Rozin et al., 1999; Shaver et al., 1987).
Disgust—contamination, physical or moral (Rozin et al., 1994, 2000).
Shame—a significant social (and perhaps moral) transgression (Keltner & Buswell, 1997).
Surprise—sudden presence of an unexpected occurrence, either positive or negative (Izard, 1991; Tomkins, 1962).

When unconscious or conscious cognitive activating appraisals detect these core circumstances, the emotion is elicited (Bowins, 2004, 2006). The core

DOI: 10.4324/b23346-12

circumstances have evolutionary fitness implications with the emotion motivating adaptive behavior (Bowins, 2006). Examples include:

Sadness: responding to loss by conserving resources, seeking new resources, or compensating in some fashion.

Fear: avoiding the threat or danger and withdrawing, or flight/fight/freeze responses if the threat or danger is intense and immediate.

Anger: addressing the violation or damage with defensive actions and/or aggressive behavior.

Disgust: withdrawing and distancing from contamination, including morally repulsive events.

Shame: responding to the social transgression with appeasement type actions.

Happiness: approaching and attempting to maintain and maximize the gain.

Interest: exploring the potential for reward to optimize resources.

Surprise: approach or withdrawal behavior depending on whether the stimulus is positive or negative.

These primary emotions quite effectively cover the range of evolutionary fitness relevant occurrences humans encountered in our 200,000- to 300,000-year evolution, motivating adaptive responses. Secondary emotions derived from combinations of primary emotions or different points on the primary emotion continuums, provide for more nuanced information and responses. For instance, contempt as a combination of anger and disgust (Rozin et al., 1999), and contentment as a variant of happiness. In the case of contempt, a person might assertively address the violation and then withdraw and for contentment maintain the status quo. The notion of emotion information processing provides a logical and rationale perspective regarding emotional functioning, helping to revise the common perception of emotions being irrational. Given the information and motivational value, emotions are genetically based in terms of the capacity to experience at least the primary ones, cognitive activating appraisals, motivation relevant to each emotion, and the capacity to perceive emotions in others.

An interesting aspect of emotions is that they are not just personal experiences but social as well: emotions are evident in facial expressions and body language (Ekman, 1972; Ekman & Friesen, 1971; Izard, 1994). Sadness yields a downcast facial expression and deflated body posture, for example. Fear provides a look of heightened alertness and muscle tension. Anger involves an intense focused expression and muscle priming for action. The question arises as to why there is the social component? Conceivably, it might be best to keep the information and motivation to oneself. The answer resides in the importance of social evolution and communication, not just for humans but we will focus on people here. If aware that another person is feeling sad, then offering assistance can set up a reciprocal situation whereby when in need the other person will help. If the person assisted is genetically related there is also the passage on one's own genes to the next generation (kin selection), assuming the assistance aids in survival and reproduction. Detecting fear in another person alerts that there is a threat or danger present, or that the person is perceiving you to be a threat, both scenarios requiring a defensive response. Anger means that the person might attack and this needs to be addressed by withdrawal, being prepared physically, and defensive or aggressive actions. On a more positive note, happiness indicates that the person is pleased by your presence or has acquired some resource that might be shared. Hence, emotions are social as well as personal. Based on the social component, we have the capacity to perceive emotions in others derived from facial expression recognition and body language, and understand the information value in regard to core circumstances. The emotion is also felt accounting for the contagion of emotions. These abilities are genetically based although refined through experience. When these social cognition capacities are significantly impaired, as with autism spectrum issues, functioning is greatly diminished (see Human Specific Cognition in the Impaired States and Processes for Mental Health chapter).

Emotion information processing, ensuing motivation, social expression, perception of emotions in others, understanding the meaning, and feeling the same emotion, has been so crucial for evolutionary fitness that it is genetically wired into us, such that it "feels" natural. It is only when impairments transpire that we really notice based on reduced functioning. Considering the significance of emotions and emotion information processing issues in clients, it naturally follows that therapists must be able to process emotions expressed by clients, and also work with their own emotional reactions as revealed in the Countertransference chapter. A key psychotherapeutic capacity derived from the spectrum of emotion information processing is empathy.

Empathy

While the term empathy gives a sense of what it is about there are many ways of interpreting it. It has been viewed as a capacity, trait, emotion, cognition, motivation, action, perspective taking, understanding, attention, appreciation, sensitivity, and in still other fashions (Elliot et al., 2018). Carl Rogers (1957) believed that empathy is one of the core therapist conditions, enabling an accurate perception of the internal frame of reference of the client along with emotions and meanings. From a psychoanalytic perspective, it is an aspect of attention opening up channels of interaction facilitating a trusting bond, and enabling the therapist to access the emotional qualities of the client's experience (Aragno, 2008). Person-centered psychotherapy and psychoanalysis are the two forms of psychotherapy placing a strong emphasis on empathy (Elliot et al., 2018), but it is generally considered to be important across all forms of psychotherapy, qualifying it as a non-specific influence (Bachar, 1998; Bowins, 2021).

Barrett-Lennard (1993) identifies three aspects of empathy including: resonance whereby the therapist resonates with the client's experiences, therapist communication of the understanding derived from the resonance, and then the client receives the therapist's empathy to feel understood. With so many ways of conceptualizing empathy and its important role in psychotherapy it is worth trying to elucidate the key aspects. A study by Kurtz and Grummon (1972) highlights the importance of this quest: the researchers applied every measure of empathy to that point in time to client perceived and tape judged empathy, finding that the measures were unrelated to each other indicating that they were assessing different variables.

Empathy most prominently is emotional if for no other reason than the feeling basis: it is impossible to have true empathy with no feeling. Returning to emotion information processing and the social aspect, the evolution of emotions includes communication via facial expressions and body language. As part of social cognition, we have the capacity to interpret facial expressions and body language, mostly unconsciously. In this regard, some emotions are easier than others with fear, sadness, anger, disgust, surprise, and happiness usually being easiest. Shame and interest are somewhat more challenging if just facial expressions are utilized as in research, but more accessible when body language is added. Of significance, this is probably why both facial expressions and body language communicate emotions: one source might not fully inform but the combination increases accuracy of perception. Demonstrating the evolutionary importance of the social aspect of emotions, the tone of a person's verbal communication can also convey emotional information. For example, we readily interpret sad, happy, interested, angry, and fearful tones in a person's speech. Difficulties perceiving emotions transpire when social cognition is impaired. When emotions are perceived in another person we infer the reason for the feeling, usually unconsciously, essentially reversing the way that emotions are triggered by cognitive activating appraisals derived from core circumstances. For instance, inferring that the person is registering a gain if happy and a loss if sad. Of course, this is all based on perceptions, as the person experiencing the emotion might perceive a gain or loss that is not really present, and the accuracy in reading emotions in others is not perfect. However, it generally works quite well in line with the evolutionary value of emotion information processing and its social aspect.

Perceiving emotions in others and unconsciously inferring the reason for it, typically yields two additional outcomes: feeling the emotion and prosocial motivation. Perceiving the emotion produces the same emotional response that the other person is experiencing (assuming that the perception is accurate), as for example seeing sadness and feeling sad, or the perception of fear producing a fearful feeling. This capacity probably follows from inferring the reason for why the other person is experiencing the emotion, because the relevant cognitive activating appraisal triggers the emotion, such as when sadness is perceived, loss is inferred, serving as a cognitive activating appraisal for sadness.

Likewise, if happiness is detected, a gain is evident, serving as a cognitive activating appraisal for a happy feeling. This entire process tends to occur naturally although some people are better at it than others, as with all capacities. This natural ability accounts for the contagion of emotions. Despite how natural it is to feel the emotions of others, two dissociative processes can interfere, the first being a psychopathic nature and the second traumatic defensive dissociation. In the Personality Disorders chapter, we looked at Antisocial Personality Disorder in terms of the evolution of deceit and enhanced dissociative capacity, enabling the person to read facial expressions and body language relevant to emotions and infer the reason, but remain emotionally detached to facilitate deception (Bowins, 2010; Intrator, 1997; Patrick et al., 1994). Psychopaths are detached from the emotions of others not due to brain damage in most instances, but because marked dissociation from the feeling state of others is necessary for this level of deceit: if the deceiver feels the suffering of the victim then their facial expressions and/or body language might inform the victim of what is transpiring, thereby compromising the deception.

Dissociation from feeling the emotions of others can also transpire with traumatic dissociation, typically occurring when a person has experienced severe trauma, the defensive response of detaching from emotional experiences reducing psychological pain. In this scenario, the person is also usually detached from emotions pertaining to their own experiences, unlike psychopaths who are aware of their own feelings and often utilize this information to adjust deceptions. For instance, if the psychopath feels good as a variant of happiness it informs that the deception is proceeding well, but frustration or anger indicates that it is not likely to work motivating a shift in the approach. Even though the traumatized person is detached from their feelings they are likely to feel remorse if made aware that their actions have hurt another person, but not the psychopath who is detached from the suffering of others. With therapy oriented to fusing dissociated aspects of the traumatic experience, those with traumatic defensive dissociation can reconnect to the feelings of others, but not the true psychopath.

Prosocial motivation naturally follows from feeling what others are experiencing, because it is like you are the one in the given circumstances. Hence, if you feel the other person's fear you want to help them reduce the threat or danger. Likewise, feeling their sadness motivates you to help manage the loss. Psychopaths who do not feel what the other person is experiencing lack this prosocial motivation, for the obvious reason that it counters the capacity to deceive and fosters remorse when the other person is deceived. Free of prosocial motivation and remorse, deception capacity to further resource acquisition is enhanced.

An interesting and debated aspect of empathy is whether or not it includes perspective taking. The position that perspective taking is not part of empathy is articulated by Stietz et al. (2019), who see the cognitive mechanisms of understanding others as not integral to empathy, and perspective taking distinct.

From the "perspective" of emotion information processing it does not appear to be either/or, but dependent on what aspect of cognitive understanding is considered. The perception of emotions in others and inferring the reasons why the person is experiencing the given feeling, provides a very robust understanding of the other person's perspective. For instance, perceiving a client's fear I know that the person is processing some threat or danger and the likelihood of anxiety is quite significant. Likewise, if I see sadness in a client it follows that the person is perceiving losses and the possibility of depression is enhanced. No verbal communication is necessary for me to take the emotional perspective of the person. Beyond emotion information processing, perspective taking is not part of empathy as we have no way of reading the thoughts of another person. What is required in this scenario is information derived from verbal communication or some other source, such as when I read a referral note for a prospective client, then I know something about the person's perspective. It might be suggested that as a therapist gets to know a client it is possible to anticipate the perspective that the client will take on occurrences, such as another romance setback. However, this capacity is based on knowledge of the client derived from emotional and non-emotional information processing, with more exposure to the client yielding better predictions of their perspective.

Hence, empathy as an emotional experience based on emotion information processing includes:

- The capacity for primary emotions (and following from this secondary emotions).
- Core circumstances for each emotion.
- Cognitive activating appraisals eliciting the emotion once the core circumstances are detected.
- Social communication of emotions in facial expressions and body language.
- Capacity to interpret emotions in others from facial expressions and body language.
- Inferring the reasons for why the emotion is experienced by the person, yielding emotion based perspective taking.
- Feeling the emotion perceived in another person.
- Prosocial motivation.

Non-emotional perspective taking is different and derived from non-emotional sources of information. Given the importance of empathy to emotional capacity the question arises as to whether or not it actually evolved? It is feasible that empathy per se did not evolve based on how it unfolds naturally from the components of emotion information processing just mentioned, but two related outcomes might have driven the evolution. First, how empathy fosters social connectedness from the sense of being understood by another person, the capacity to experience the emotional perspective of others, and prosocial motivation, with social connectedness crucial given our social evolution.

Second, how the trust that empathy fosters can set up reciprocal relationships that were a key factor in human evolution, due to the value of exchanging needed resources.

Empathy enables the therapist to connect with and understand the emotional world of clients. This capacity extends across all therapies and mental health conditions as a key non-specific factor. Empathy also fosters additional therapist-based emotional capacities including: compassion, support, involvement, and the therapist's role in the therapeutic alliance. Given the powerful impact of empathy in the emotional aspects of therapy, it is almost inconceivable that it would not influence outcomes in a positive fashion. Indeed, research supports the role of empathy in robust psychotherapy outcomes. Elliot et al. (2018) reviewed 82 studies finding that empathy generally accounts for 9% of the variance in psychotherapy outcomes with a moderate effect size. The results held across various theoretical perspectives and presenting problems. Nienhuis et al. (2018) conducted a meta-analysis of 53 studies examining empathy, genuineness, and the therapeutic alliance. They found that the therapeutic alliance was significantly associated with perceptions of therapist empathy and genuineness, and that empathy and genuineness overlapped when rated by the same person. Indicating how significant the therapist's emotional involvement derived from empathy is, Peluso and Freund (2018) examined the association between both therapist and client expression of emotions and psychotherapy outcome, finding that both were significant with the client's contribution somewhat greater, understandable given that the client is the person experiencing difficulties. Therapist empathic ability fosters a healthy therapeutic alliance, likely accounting for why high-empathy therapists have better success rates regardless of theoretical orientation, whereas low-empathy therapists experience higher dropout and relapse rates and less positive change (Moyers & Miller, 2013). Watson et al. (2014) found that client perceptions of therapist empathy are important, these perceptions linked to significant improvements in attachment insecurity and functioning, and significant decreases in negative self-treatment.

Various problems addressed by psychotherapy seem to respond to empathy, such as alcohol issues. Moyers et al. (2016) audio recorded 38 therapists working with 700 clients undergoing a behavioral intervention for problem drinking. Their analysis of the data revealed that 11% of the variance in drinking was accounted for by therapists and that empathy was the most significant contributor. Focusing on depression, McClintock et al. (2018) examined 56 clients undergoing psychotherapy for depression by 6 students. The experiencing of therapist empathy early in treatment contributed to the therapeutic alliance, in turn facilitating improvement in depression symptoms. Another study revealing the positive impact of therapist empathy early in treatment is that by Hara et al. (2017), in this instance for generalized anxiety. They studied 43 therapist-client dyads over 15 sessions of cognitive behavioral therapy, finding that greater early empathy was associated with better mid-treatment homework compliance, and this compliance was related to lower post-treatment worry (Hara et al., 2017).

These research results support the robust contribution of therapist empathy to psychotherapy outcomes across various types of therapy and mental health conditions. Empathy provides a portal to the emotional experience of the client, and connects the client and therapist in a positive way contributing to the therapeutic alliance. Limited empathy, or none as with psychopaths, greatly impedes the progress of psychotherapy, whereas a solid capacity fosters good outcomes.

EMOTIONAL STABILITY

The emotional stability of a client is relevant to psychotherapy outcomes, as discussed at various points in the Client Influences section. Equally important in all likelihood is that of the therapist, although this topic receives little attention relative to client emotional stability. An emotionally unstable therapist will react too strongly to client actions, including transference and immature defense mechanisms expression, thereby impairing the therapeutic relationship. Assuming that therapy does continue, the client will internalize emotional volatility instead of robust regulation over emotions, contributing to further emotional difficulties that will impact negatively on therapy and the therapeutic alliance. Hence, it is very important for the therapist to be emotionally stable. There are various sources of therapist emotional instability including use of immature psychological defense mechanisms, deficient emotion regulation, excessive reactivity, and lack of confidence, many of these representing impaired states and processes for mental health, covered in the chapter of that name.

Regular use of immature psychological defense mechanisms results in emotional instability, whereas mature defense mechanism use provides for emotional stability. Acting out, splitting, idealization/devaluation, projection, and projective identification, for instance, result in a rollercoaster of emotions more characteristic of clients with personality disorders, and most prominently Borderline Personality Disorder (see the Personality Disorders chapter), than therapists. Where I have heard of this problem with therapists is when a person who suffered abuse in early life decides to be a therapist, but has not progressed sufficiently in their own treatment. Making matters worse, countertransference reactions to clients derived from the therapist's trauma history can intensify the use of immature defenses. Replacing these immature defenses with mature ones such as sublimation, altruism, positive anticipation, humor, and suppression, will greatly bolster emotion regulation (see Borderline Personality Disorder in the Personality Disorders chapter for further information). Fortunately, this transition occurs with longer term psychotherapy of different forms and so can definitely be corrected.

Deficient emotion regulation can arise from various sources, and quite prominently, overuse of immature psychological defense mechanisms, and so by shifting defenses from immature to mature, emotion regulation is advanced. Additional approaches can be applied including reframing perspectives contributing to excessively intense negative emotions which harnesses the power of emotion information processing, absorption in positive pursuits to replace negative emotions with positive ones, and focusing on components of emotion regulation identified by Gratz and Roemer (2004): awareness of emotional responses, clarity of emotional responses, acceptance of emotional responses, access to emotion regulation strategies perceived as effective, controlling impulses when experiencing negative emotions, and engaging in goal-directed behaviors when experiencing negative emotions (see Psychological Regulation in the Impaired States and Processes for Mental Health chapter).

Excessive reactivity naturally contributes to emotional instability, and is derived from a high level on the neurotic-emotionally stable dimension of normal personality, part of the Big 5 model of personality by Costa and McCrae (1992) (see the Personality Disorders chapter). As discussed in the Personality Disorders chapter, neurotic is simply a label that should be replaced by reactivity. Anyone rating high in reactivity will be less emotionally stable and have greater challenges with emotion regulation. To moderate excessive reactivity application of the SUPPRESS-THINK-RESPOND technique, covered in the Resistance and Noncompliance chapter, is important: suppress (a mature defense mechanism) the immediate response, apply balanced thought, and with this input respond. It is a simple technique that can help a person gain control over a highly reactive nature.

Poor confidence can also contribute to emotional instability, and this usually occurs in the context of a therapist with limited experience, perhaps still in training, who is quite self-critical and less self-accepting. Add in clients utilizing immature defenses, such as splitting and idealization/devaluation, and negative transference, and it is easy to see how and why low confidence and negative emotions transpire in self-critical inexperienced therapists. With any complex skill such as psychotherapy it is normal to be somewhat insecure initially, but if a person is self-critical relatively minor mistakes will be blown out of proportion and impair confidence. As covered in the Impaired States and Processes for Mental Health chapter under Self-Acceptance, it is important to shift from a self-critical stance to acceptance of the inevitability of mistakes and learning from them, rather than beating oneself up and in essence wielding a sledgehammer against the foundation of one's being. Understood as a repetitive maladaptive pattern of behavior, self-criticism must be consciously addressed ongoing to gradually replace this dysfunctional pattern with one of self-support bolstering self-concept, self-esteem, and hence self-acceptance. Although the amorphous nature of psychotherapy lends itself to low confidence in the context of self-criticisms, a helpful concept is the notion that with approximately 10,000 hours of experience in anything complex you are an expert, with brain synapses wired to facilitate ease of applying the skill, and with ongoing devotion to psychotherapy those hours will come. As an aside, a benefit of focusing on states and processes for mental health, such as self-acceptance, is that it provides a clear across therapy and trans-diagnostic approach to psychotherapy countering the seemingly amorphous nature of it.

WORKING WITH EMOTIONAL FACTORS

Impaired therapist emotional capacity and stability are very detrimental to psychotherapy outcomes and do need to be addressed. Of profound significance, the capacity for empathy is a must with all the components of emotion information processing in place, enabling the client's emotions to be felt and the reasons for them inferred. Emotion information processing is an evolutionary based capacity and it comes naturally for most of us, but can be greatly limited with impaired social cognition. This is why people with social cognition problems do not make for good psychotherapists, and can really only function at all with highly manualized approaches that can also be delivered by computer interfaces. I realize that some people might object to this, but psychotherapy is more for the client than the therapist, and people who have a limitation that is difficult if not impossible to overcome will jeopardize psychotherapy outcomes to the detriment of the client. You would not want a mostly blind dentist working on your teeth, and likewise should not want a therapist who is unable to be empathic. If the social cognition limitations are minor, such as struggling to read facial expressions for harder to decipher emotions or fully grasping complex social-emotional scenarios such as sarcasm, then practice and learning can ramp up these capacities, fostering stronger empathy. For example, utilizing online facial expression programs to practice emotion recognition and reading more about emotion information processing.

If the empathy limitation resides in dissociation from the feelings of others then there is a major problem. A psychopathic nature will be disastrous for clients and psychotherapy outcomes, given that this evolved mechanism utilizing dissociation is designed to foster deceit and manipulation. It is no wonder that successful psychotherapists are high on empathy and low on a psychopathic nature. If the dissociation from the feelings of others is due to defensive dissociation related to trauma, then the prospective therapist needs to be a client first before attempting to be a therapist, and only venture to this career if able to fuse the dissociated aspects of the trauma. With robust empathy, other emotion related capacities, such as compassion, support, involvement, and the therapist's role in the therapeutic alliance are advanced assisting in the progress of psychotherapy.

Emotional instability is easier to address and remedy than empathy problems. Overuse of immature defense mechanisms typically requires longer term therapy, assisted by active learning of mature psychological defenses. Immature defenses contribute to emotion regulation problems, and so by addressing the defense mechanism issue regulation over emotions will improve. The additional steps of absorption in positive pursuits to replace negative emotions with positive emotions, and the strategies identified by Gratz and Roemer (2004), consisting of awareness of emotional responses, clarity of emotional responses, acceptance of emotional responses, access to emotion regulation strategies perceived as effective, controlling impulses when experiencing negative emotions, and engaging in goal-directed behaviors when experiencing negative emotions, can be very helpful when it comes to regulating negative emotions.

A highly reactive nature contributes to emotional instability, but by applying the three-step technique of suppressing immediate responses, rethinking the situation briefly, and then responding on this basis, excessive reactions are transformed into less reactive and more constructive responses. In this regard, think of politicians who either naturally learn or are trained to inhibit their immediate response and rapidly think of the best response, with the momentary pause barely noticeable and often suggesting that the question or prompt is worthy of thought. The possibility of a reactive and negative response diminishing support is replaced by impactful responses voters want to hear. Strong emotional reactivity is not always a negative either, given that it enhances sensitivity to low amplitude emotions of clients that a low reactive therapist might miss. The key is to regulate the inclination to verbally and behaviorally respond excessively to the input. Emotional instability derived from inexperience, often combined with self-criticisms, is quite straightforward to address by replacing the dysfunctional pattern of self-criticisms with self-support fostering good self-concept, self-esteem, and hence self-acceptance.

SUMMARY NOTE

Both impaired empathy (and the emotion related influences following from this crucial capacity) and emotional instability, make for a very limited therapist, such that psychotherapy outcomes will be severely compromised. With robust emotional capacities and most significantly empathy, and emotional stability, a therapist advances psychotherapy outcomes for clients. Therefore, it is crucial for prospective therapists and those already practicing to appreciate emotional factors and respond appropriately to limitations.

REFERENCES

Aragno, A. (2008). The language of empathy: An Analysis of its constitution, development, and role in psychoanalytic listening. *Journal of the American Psychoanalytic Association*, *56*(3), 713–740.

Bachar, E. (1998). Psychotherapy—an active agent: Assessing the effectiveness of psychotherapy and its curative factors. *Israel Journal of Psychiatry and Related Sciences*, *35*(2), 128–135.

Barrett-Lennard, G. T. (1993). The phases and focus of empathy. *British Journal of Medical Psychology*. https://doi.org/10.1111/j.2044-8341.1993.tb01722.x

Beck, A. (1991). Cognitive therapy: A 30-year retrospective. *American Psychologist*, *46*(4), 368–375.

Boucher, J., & Carlson, G. (1980). Recognition of facial expression in three cultures. *Journal of Cross-Cultural Psychology*, *11*, 263–280.

Bowins, B. E. (2004). Psychological defense mechanisms: A new perspective. *American Journal of Psychoanalysis, 64*, 1–26.

Bowins, B. E. (2006). How psychiatric treatments can enhance psychological defense mechanisms. *American Journal of Psychoanalysis, 66*, 173–194.

Bowins, B. E. (2010). Personality disorders: A dimensional defense mechanism approach. *American Journal of Psychotherapy, 64*(2), 153–169.

Bowins, B. E. (2021). *States and processes for mental health: Advancing psychotherapy effectiveness.* Academic Press.

Costa, P. T., & McCrae, R. R. (1992). *Revised NEO personality (NEO-PI-R) and NEO five factor inventory (NEO-FFI). Professional journal manual.* Psychological Assessment Resources.

Ekman, P. (1972). *Emotions in the human face.* Cambridge University Press.

Ekman, P., & Friesen, W. (1971). Constants across cultures in the face and emotion. *Journal of Personality and Social Psychology, 17*, 124–129.

Eley, T., & Stevenson, J. (2000). Specific life events and chronic experiences differentially associated with depression and anxiety in young twins. *Journal of Abnormal Child Psychology, 28*(4), 383–394.

Elliot, R., Bohart, A. C., Watson, J. C., & Murphy, D. (2018). Therapist empathy and client outcome: An updated meta-analysis. *Psychotherapy, 55*(4), 399–410.

Finlay-Jones, R., & Brown, G. (1981). Types of stressful life event and the onset of anxiety and depressive disorders. *Psychological Medicine, 11*, 803–815.

Gratz, K. L., & Roemer, L. (2004). Multidimensional assessment of emotion regulation and dysregulation: Development, factor structure, and initial validation of the difficulties in emotion regulation scale. *Journal of Psychopathology and Behavioral Assessment, 26*, 41–54.

Hara, K. M., Aviram, A., Constantino, M. J., Westra, H. A., & Antony, M. M. (2017). Therapist empathy, homework compliance, and outcome in cognitive behavioral therapy for generalized anxiety disorder: Partitioning within-and between-therapist effects. *Cognitive Behavioral Therapy, 46*(5), 375–390.

Intrator, J. (1997). A brain imaging (single photon emission computerized tomography) study of semantic and affective processing in psychopaths. *Biological Psychiatry, 42*, 96–103.

Izard, C. (1991). *The psychology of emotions.* Plenum Press.

Izard, C. (1994). Innate and universal facial expressions: Evidence from developmental and cross-cultural research. *Psychological Bulletin, 115*(2), 288–299.

Keltner, D., & Buswell, B. (1997). Embarrassment: Its distinct form and appeasement functions. *Psychological Bulletin, 122*(3), 250–270.

Kurtz, R. R., & Grummon, D. L. (1972). Different approaches to the measurement of therapist empathy and their relationship to therapy outcomes. *Journal of Consulting and Clinical Psychology, 39*(1), 106–115.

McClintock, A. S., Anderson, T., Patterson, C. L., & Wing, E. H. (2018). Early psychotherapeutic empathy, alliance, and client outcome: Preliminary evidence of indirect effects. *Journal of Clinical Psychology, 74*(6), 839–848.

Moyers, T. B., Houck, J., Rice, S. L., Longabaugh, R., & Miller, W. R. (2016). Therapist empathy, combined behavioral intervention, and alcohol outcomes in the COMBINE research project. *Journal of Consulting and Clinical Psychology, 84*(3), 221–229.

Moyers, T. B., & Miller, W. R. (2013). Is low therapist empathy toxic? *Psychology of Addictive Behaviors, 27*(3), 878–884.

Nienhuis, J. B., Owen, J., Valentine, J. C., Black, S. W., Halford, T. C., Parazak, S. E., et al. (2018). Therapeutic alliance, empathy, and genuineness in individual adult psychotherapy: A meta-analytic review. *Psychotherapy Research, 28*(4), 593–605.

Patrick, C., Cuthbert, B., & Lang, P. (1994). Emotion in the criminal psychopath: Fear image processing. *Journal of Abnormal Psychology*, *103*(3), 523–534.

Peluso, P. R., & Freund, R. R. (2018). Therapist and client emotional expression and psychotherapy outcomes: A meta-analysis. *Psychotherapy (Chic)*, *55*(4), 461–472.

Rogers, C. R. (1957). The necessary and sufficient conditions of therapeutic personality change. *Journal of Consulting Psychology*, *21*(2), 95–103.

Rozin, P., Haidt, J., & McCauley, C. (2000). Disgust. *Handbook of emotions* (2nd ed.) The Guilford Press.

Rozin, P., Lowery, L., & Ebert, R. (1994). Varieties of disgust faces and the structure of disgust. *Journal of Personality and Social Psychology*, *66*(5), 870–881.

Rozin, P., Lowery, L., Imada, S., & Haidt, J. (1999). The CAD triad hypothesis: A mapping between three moral emotions (contempt, anger, disgust) and three moral codes (community, autonomy, divinity). *Journal of Personality and Social Psychology*, *76*(4), 574–586.

Shaver, P., Schwartz, J., Kirson, D., & O'Connor, C. (1987). Emotion knowledge: Further exploration of a prototype approach. *Journal of Personality and Social Psychology*, *52*(6), 1086–1091.

Stietz, J., Jauk, E., Krach, S., & Kanske, P. (2019). Dissociating empathy from perspective-taking: Evidence from intra- and inter-individual differences research. *Frontiers in Psychology*. https://doi.org/10.3389/fpsyt.2019.00126

Tomkins, S. (1962). *Affect, imagery, consciousness: The positive effects (Vol. 1)*. Springer.

Watson, J. C., Steckley, P. L., & McMullen, E. J. (2014). The role of empathy in promoting change. *Psychotherapy Research*. https://doi.org/10.1080/10503307.2013.802823

Chapter 11

PERSONALITY FACTORS

Personality encompasses many qualities that have the potential to influence the capacity of a psychotherapist, and hence progress with psychotherapy. As covered in the Personality Disorders chapter, normal personality as typically understood utilizing the trait approach, is somewhat different than abnormal personality. Most research examining therapist personality factors excludes personality disorders due, firstly, to how it is unlikely that a practicing psychotherapist will have a full-fledged personality disorder, and secondly, how the current diagnostic approach is either/or with a certain number of criteria required to yield a personality disorder diagnoses. However, personality disorders can be conceptualized as extreme and enduring expressions of normal psychological defense processes (Bowins, 2010, 2016): see the Personality Disorders chapter for information regarding the defense mechanism perspective. Understood as a continuum of normal defensive processes, abnormal personality is applicable to a discussion of therapist personality factors. Hence, we will look at abnormal and normal personality factors pertinent to therapists.

ABNORMAL PERSONALITY

Although it is highly unlikely that a therapist will suffer from an intense degree of any personality disorder, somewhat higher expressions along the continuum are viable for Avoidant, Narcissistic, Dependent, Obsessive-Compulsive, and Borderline personality disorders. As covered in the Emotional Factors chapter, Antisocial Personality Disorder is incompatible with being a therapist, and it is unlikely that a person with very low empathic ability will try to become a therapist or function well enough to continue. I will now indicate how the given personality disorder issue can impact adversely on the therapist's capacity to function effectively, with a brief coverage of how to address the problem; for a full coverage of the given personality disorder, including treatment, see the Personality Disorders chapter.

DOI: 10.4324/b23346-13

Avoidant Personality Disorder

Avoidance of scenarios that are not objectively threatening that offer the potential for reward is dysfunctional in any context. How this can materialize for therapists is failure to address anxiety provoking topics that have the potential to help the client. For example, an avoidant therapist might feel uncomfortable discussing sexual orientation or sexual performance issues, and avoid the topic, or communicate a lack of comfort in facial expressions and body language if raised by the client. I mention these examples because they are the most common topics clients have expressed representing difficulties for some therapists they have tried to work with, and appreciate my comfort level in discussing the issue in a non-judgmental fashion. Any topic that has personal relevance to the therapist, such that it elicits anxiety, will be avoided if avoidance problems exist. If the client suffers from the given issue, then therapy will not progress well. Fortunately, if the therapist recognizes the problem resolution transpires by facing anxiety provoking topics in a graded fashion from least to most feared, a strategy that almost invariably lessens the anxiety. Avoidance reinforces anxiety whereas approach reduces it. Ongoing approach in terms of addressing anxiety provoking themes not only reduces anxiety but increases competence, and serves as an example to clients who experience anxiety and avoidance problems.

Narcissistic Personality Disorder

Excessive compensation for vulnerabilities represents a risk for therapists, because the over compensation can interfere with empathy and the therapeutic alliance. For instance, if the therapist is insecure regarding knowledge and over compensates by insisting that their perspective is correct, the client's emotional perspective will not be processed. The client might be presenting how depression was experienced and the therapist strongly asserts that this manifestation does not characterize depression, instead of appreciating that the client's experience is what matters, even if it does not fit with the therapist's conceptualization of the illness. By remedying vulnerabilities and proactively inhibiting intense compensation, the degree of narcissism can be reduced to normal levels indicated by reasonable compensation for insecurities. The therapist's capacity to truly listen to clients will then be strengthened.

Dependent Personality Disorder

Given our social evolution we all rely on others, but excessive reliance compromises independent functioning, and therapists have to be able to function independently. I have noted this problem with insecure and anxiety prone therapists, who have trouble making diagnostic and therapeutic decisions on their own, excessively seeking advice from other therapists and requesting too many consultations. Psychotherapy is usually not a team endeavor involving regular exchanges with colleagues, and therapists have to function independently. While it is fine and adaptive to discuss complex cases with colleagues, compromised independence communicates insecurity to clients that can impair their trust in the therapist. If the client has dependency issues, then it also reinforces the problem, as the therapist's insecurity and excessive dependence are internalized. Dependent personality problems can be rectified by approaching scenarios that elicit insecure feelings and dependent behavior in a graded fashion, while reducing self-criticisms and increasing self-approval. For instance, instead of criticizing oneself for errors when a new approach to therapy is tried, accept that we all make mistakes and learn from them. This approach bolsters therapeutic skills, communicates confidence to the client assisting in trust of the therapist, and serves as a template for independent behavior that can be internalized by the client.

Obsessive-Compulsive Personality Disorder

Compulsive type behavior does help manage anxiety, but excessive compulsiveness reduces flexibility and adaptability which is crucial for therapists if they are to be effective. For example, overly focusing on the client attending sessions right on time, and strongly critiquing lateness, might impede an exploration of the client's feelings of being ineffectual and the passive-aggressive behavior arising from such feelings. Even excessive adherence to a manualized psychotherapy approach will ironically impede the progress of psychotherapy, because issues always arise that cannot be scripted and flexibly addressing these concerns assists with the given problem, while fostering a solid therapeutic alliance. If excessive compulsivity is present, then refraining from acting compulsively drawing on the technique of exposure and response prevention can reduce anxiety, lessen the compulsive behavior, and increase flexibility. In the example of the therapist who overly adheres to punctual attendance, refrain from criticizing the occurrence and instead openly explore the reasons behind it.

Borderline Personality Disorder

Reliance on immature psychological defenses, which is prominent with this personality disorder, compromises many aspects of a therapist's performance, and contributes greatly to emotional instability (see the Emotional Factors chapter). It is not difficult to imagine how projecting negative aspects of oneself onto the client, idealizing and then devaluing the person, acting out countertransference, only identifying with certain emotions felt when they are incited in the client (projective identification), and the like, will prevent any progress in therapy. While it is rare to encounter pronounced Borderline Personality Disorder in a therapist, more minor degrees do occur often in the context of a therapist traumatized in their youth who adopts this career. Engaging in longer term psychotherapy, particularly with a focus on psychological defense mechanisms, can shift the profile from immature to mature defenses, with suppression, humor, sublimation, altruism, and positive anticipation capable of being consciously learned. Emotion regulation is advanced, and this change will assist clients in internalizing solid regulation of emotions.

NORMAL PERSONALITY

The list of normal personality traits linked to effective therapist performance is extensive. In a review, Ackerman and Hilsenroth (2003) cite flexible, honest, respectful, trustworthy, confident, warm, interested, and open contributing positively to the therapeutic alliance. Benjamin (2015) emphasizes curiosity and creativity in line with the artistic side of psychotherapy. Focusing on psychoanalytic therapy, Goldstein and Suzuki (2015) indicate that authenticity is important, expressed in unformulated insight oriented or even simple acknowledgment comments, demonstrating that the therapist is willing to speak aloud without screening. Based on his own experience as an analyst and a review of the literature, Greben (1977) lists empathy and concern, caring and protectiveness, warmth, therapeutic forcefulness, friendliness and respectfulness, positive expectations, freedom from despair, and reliability. Many of the various personality traits indicated can be subsumed under virtue and prosocial, although clustering is a challenge. Psychologically minded is another important trait, identified by Farber et al. (2005) in a review of why people become therapists, very important given that psychologically minded provides a good fit with this career option, and if limited there will be a major impediment to psychotherapy outcomes from the start. In addition, psychological mindedness encompasses traits that favor success as a psychotherapist such as insightful, awareness and appreciation of psychological problems, generation of solutions to psychological issues, emphasis on emotions, and understanding various perspectives.

The normal personality traits identified to this point are quite diffuse, although many can be subsumed under virtue, prosocial, and psychologically minded. What about personality traits that characterize people generally? In this regard, the 5-factor model (FFM) of temperament/personality, that has come to be known as the "Big 5" (Costa & McCrae, 1992), stands out, with the five bipolar dimensions of extraversion-introversion, neurotic-emotionally stable, open-closed to experience, agreeable-antagonism, and conscientious-negligence. In the Personality Disorders chapter, it was mentioned that the names are labels that do not necessarily indicate the true nature of the given dimension, and where this is problematic is with the neurotic-emotionally stable one that probably is a reactivity dimension. Low reactivity equates with emotional stability and high reactivity aligns with neurotic, which is actually quite a negative label. Hence, we will consider this dimension as low to high reactivity.

Limited research does examine how therapist ratings on the Big 5 influence psychotherapy. Chapman et al. (2009) examined 34 training therapists administering the NEO-Five Factor Inventory (NEO-FFI), and applied ratings of both client and therapist assessments of the therapeutic alliance. Introversion-extroversion and conscientious-negligence did not have any impact (Chapman et al., 2009). High openness produced lower client ratings of the alliance, that the researchers surmise might have been related to eccentric qualities of the therapist that are more challenging for clients to align with (Chapman et al., 2009). They indicate that moderate levels of openness produced better ratings by clients. Higher levels of "neuroticism" yielded better client ratings of the therapeutic alliance, that the researchers attributed to the therapist experiencing more negative emotions enabling the client to identify with the therapist, but indicate that "neuroticism" was not that high in the sample. Higher agreeableness was associated with lower trainee ratings of the therapeutic alliance, but the link was weak. This unusual result might have been due to how agreeable people are often humble yielding lower self-ratings (Chapman et al., 2009). Another study found that openness and neuroticism (reactivity) scores were in the high range for 49 student therapists, while the other Big 5 personality traits were average (Boswell et al., 2009). In the Ackerman and Hilsenroth (2003) review mentioned earlier, openness emerged as a personal attribute that positively influenced the therapeutic alliance. In a study of cognitive behavioral therapists, agreeableness was positively associated with clinical skill (Branson & Shafran, 2015).

Examining the reverse scenario—how practice as a psychotherapist influences personality—Grunberger and Laireiter (2013) conducted an online survey of 152 therapists with personality assessments, including the NEO-FFI. The changes were retrospective limiting the validity, but they found that agreeableness, openness, and self-confidence increased while neuroticism decreased. These results do make sense because experience as a therapist improves the capacity to work with people improving agreeableness, one becomes more open to discussing a variety of issues, and from the learning and self-knowledge develops more confidence, while reactivity (neuroticism) diminishes with repetition and confidence.

Some of the Big 5 personality traits (Costa & McCrae, 1992) do seem to align with success as a psychotherapist, one being openness given that the facets contributing to it include imagination, artistic interests, depth of emotions, willingness to experiment, intellectual curiosity, and tolerance for diversity. Imagination helps a therapist envision the client's life, depth of emotions will foster empathy and prosocial motivation, psychotherapy is aided by experimentation and intellectual curiosity given the variety of issues and solutions required, and many different types of people and scenarios are encountered making tolerance of diversity important. Agreeableness also seems to align with success as a psychotherapist based on the facets of trust in others, sincerity, altruism, compliance, modesty, and sympathy. If you do not trust people it is difficult to engage with them as a therapist must. The other facets increase the clients trust in the therapist fostering an optimal therapeutic alliance. In contrast, distrust, insincere, self-focused, lack of flexibility, conceited, and uncaring characterizing a disagreeable personality, will clearly hinder the therapeutic alliance and the success of psychotherapy. Conscientiousness is a key factor in success generally regardless of the endeavor, and the facets underlying it help explain why: sense of competence, orderliness, sense of responsibility, achievement striving, self-discipline, and deliberateness. Each ensures devotion to the given task and solid follow-through (perseverance), very important when the mental health of clients is at stake. High reactivity (neuroticism) is important given that this personality profile involves anxiety, anger/hostility, moodiness, self-indulgence, and sensitivity to stress, impeding progress with psychotherapy when high, whereas more moderate levels ensure that the therapist can detect and respond to lower intensity emotions in the client and themselves. Extraversion is not quite as straightforward with some of the facets assisting in being a therapist, such as warmth, assertiveness, and positive emotions, and others like excitement seeking, activity level, and gregariousness not as clear cut, although not obviously detrimental. The individual facets of the Big 5 traits then do help to explain why openness to experience, agreeableness, and conscientiousness foster success as a therapist, and why high reactivity is likely detrimental. Regarding extroversion, it might be the case that a more moderate level assisting with warmth, assertiveness, and positive emotions is beneficial, but too high levels might impede the one-to-one nature of most psychotherapy relationships and detract from introspection.

Most of the limited research examining normal personality traits in therapists focuses on the Big 5, but a large-scale study conducted by Peter et al. (2017) involving 1,027 psychotherapists from Germany, Austria, and Switzerland, applied the Personality Style and Disorder Inventory (PSDI-5), an instrument that measures personality styles derived from the DSM-5 and ICD-10 personality disorders classification systems. Results were compared to a normative PSDI-5 sample of 3,392 individuals. One finding that counters the seemingly popular notion of therapists having mental health problems, was that on 12/14 scales the therapists scored below previously established population norms. Therapists ratings also indicated very low levels of willful/paranoid, spontaneous/borderline, reserved/schizoid, and ambitious/narcissistic (Peter et al., 2017). Willful/paranoid indicates a need to protect oneself and interpret others actions negatively. Spontaneous/borderline captures intense and unstable expression of emotions. Reserved/schizoid refers to impaired expression of emotions and intensity of expression. Ambitious/narcissistic indicates a sense of being very special and grandiose. These four traits, which are bordering on the personality disorder range, clearly make for a poor therapist, and low levels on them as found in their sample align with success as a therapist, even though the researchers did not evaluate therapist performance (Peter et al., 2017). Of relevance to the nature of personality disorders, personality trait research underlying the PSDI is based on what the DSM personality disorder categories provide, and consequently map onto this system too well, in contrast to applying factor analysis to numerous personality relevant adjectives not derived from any one system (Trull & Durrett, 2005).

Personality is expressed in behavior, dress, and also décor including that of the therapist's office, the latter leading Nasar and Devlin (2011) to assess whether features of on-campus therapy offices influence perceptions of therapist qualities. Thirty photographs of psychotherapist offices initially assessed for softness/personalization and order, were presented to university students who rated the quality of care expected in each office, and in another study, how qualified, bold, and friendly they expected the therapist to be. Perceived quality of care, comfort, therapist boldness, qualifications, and the likelihood of choosing the therapist, increased with both higher softness/personalization and order ratings of the office. Friendliness ratings improved only with higher softness/personalization. This study is unique and interesting because discussions of the role of therapist's personality in the success of psychotherapy typically rely on therapist traits, and not what expressions of personality suggest. How a therapist structures and decorates their office, assuming they have the option of doing so, does communicate information about the therapist's personality. My office includes photographs I have taken underwater, as a favorite activity is scuba diving and underwater photography, expressing my openness to experience, and clients seem to like it finding the pictures soothing, perhaps creating an expectation that I will sooth their suffering. It is then worthwhile for therapists to put some thought and effort into how their office is decorated.

Regarding what therapists can do to improve normal personality traits, at one level the answer might be relatively little in the sense that many of these traits, such as the Big 5, are genetically based and so do tend to persist. For example, people do not change radically in regard to openness to experience, conscientiousness, extraversion, agreeableness, and reactivity. However, as the results of the Grunberger and Laireiter (2013) study examining how personality changes with experience as a therapist show, there appear to be positive shifts with agreeableness, openness, and self-confidence increasing and neuroticism (reactivity) decreasing, meaning that simply practicing your craft over time will help. Adopting a persona of virtue, prosocial actions, and psychological mindedness might also assist in advancing such traits, given that roles including that of professional therapist are quite powerful in shaping behavior and expectations in oneself and others. This entails a conscious consideration and self-evaluation of traits including: flexible, honest, respectful, trustworthy, confident, warm, interested, open, curious, creative, authentic, caring and protective, assertive, friendly, positive, reliable, insightful, awareness and appreciation of psychological problems, generation of solutions to psychological issues, emphasis on emotions, and understanding various perspectives. Efforts to bolster any of these traits that are deficient through application and practice will help advance a therapist's effectiveness, while persistent deficiencies will impair performance. If the number of such traits seems overwhelming, thinking in terms of virtue, prosocial, and psychologically minded will provide a more manageable focus with the specific traits flowing from these umbrella characteristics. As the Nasar and Devlin (2011) study reveals, even paying attention to office décor is important in communicating personality traits to clients which will help shape their expectations, although the best scenario here is an office that authentically reflects positive features of your true nature.

SUMMARY NOTE

As quite fixed features of the therapist relative to skills (see the Skill Factors chapter), personality does have a very persistent influence on the therapeutic alliance and psychotherapy outcomes. While full-fledged personality disorders are unlikely in therapists, somewhat higher expressions on the continuums of Avoidant, Narcissistic, Dependent, Obsessive-Compulsive, and Borderline personality disorders can be an issue, and will impede the progress of psychotherapy. Fortunately, these issues can be remedied by the strategies outlined, which essentially entail normalizing behavior on the given personality disorder continuum. A wide variety of normal personality traits that somewhat fit under virtue, prosocial, and psychologically minded do enhance the success of psychotherapy, and can be improved by a conscious focus on the given traits and applying them to the therapist role. Regarding "Big 5" traits, simply experience practicing psychotherapy will advance the most relevant ones for success as a psychotherapist, including openness and agreeableness, with less reactivity. Hence, even though personality traits are quite fixed compared to skills, detrimental ones can definitely be improved to enhance progress with psychotherapy, whereas personality deficits not attended to will impede outcomes.

REFERENCES

Ackerman, S. J., & Hilsenroth, M. J. (2003). A review of therapist characteristics and techniques positively impacting on the therapeutic alliance. *Clinical Psychology Review, 23*(1), 1–33.

Benjamin, L. S. (2015). The arts, crafts, and sciences of psychotherapy. *Journal of Clinical Psychology, 71*(11), 1070–1082.

Boswell, J. F., Castonguay, L. G., & Pincus, A. L. (2009). Trainee theoretical orientation: Profiles and potential predictors. *Journal of Psychotherapy Integration, 19*, 291–312.

Bowins, B. E. (2010). Personality disorders: A dimensional defense mechanism approach. *American Journal of Psychotherapy, 64*(2), 153–169.

Bowins, B. E. (2016). *Mental illness defined: Continuums, regulation, and defense.* Routledge.

Branson, A., & Shafran, R. (2015). Therapist characteristics and their effect on training outcomes; what counts? *Behavioral and Cognitive Psychotherapy, 43*(3), 374–380.

Chapman, B. P., Talbot, N., Tatman, A. W., & Brition, P. C. (2009). Personality traits and the working alliance in psychotherapy trainees: An organizing role for the five factor model? *Journal of Social and Clinical Psychology, 28*(5), https://doi.org/10.1521/jscp.2009.28.5.577

Costa, P. T., & McCrae, R. R. (1992). *Revised NEO personality (NEO-PI-R) and NEO five factor inventory (NEO-FFI) professional journal manual*. Psychological Assessment Resources.

Farber, B. A., Manevich, I., Metzger, J., & Saypol, E. (2005). Choosing psychotherapy as a career; why did we cross that road? *Journal of Clinical Psychology, 61*(8), 1009–1031.

Goldstein, G., & Suzuki, J. Y. (2015). The analyst's authenticity: "If you see something, say something". *Journal of Clinical Psychology, 71*(5), 451–456.

Greben, S. E. (1977). On being therapeutic. *Canadian Psychiatric Association Journal, 22*(7), 371–380.

Grunberger, T., & Laireiter, A. R. (2013). Between growth and isolation—The influence of therapy on the experience and the personality of therapists. *Psychotherapy and Psychosomatics, 64*(1), 28–34.

Nasar, J. L., & Devlin, A. S. (2011). Impressions of psychotherapists' offices. *Journal of Counselling Psychology, 58*(3), 310–320.

Peter, B., Bobel, E., Hagl, M., Richter, M., & Kazen, M. (2017). Personality styles of German-speaking psychotherapists differ from a norm, and male psychotherapists differ from their female colleagues. *Frontiers in Psychology*. https://doi.org/10.3389/fpsyg.2017.00840

Trull, T. J., & Durrett, C. A. (2005). Categorical and dimensional models of personality disorder. *Annual Review of Clinical Psychology, 1*, 355–380.

Chapter 12

SKILL FACTORS

Compared to personality factors, skill factors can be adopted and modified relatively quickly. However, some personality traits can be modified with reasonable ease while certain skills require a great deal of effort to master. For instance, the personality trait of agreeableness can be advanced by listening and accepting client perspectives, while learning the skill of appropriate responsiveness to client issues does take some effort to master, at least in those with limited capacity. Some psychotherapy skills yoke to personality traits, such as how openness to experience favors flexibly adjusting to client needs, and moderate reactivity facilitates appropriate responsiveness. Emotional factors, and prominently empathy, also contribute to skills required by psychotherapists. With an awareness that psychotherapy skills are linked to personality and emotional factors, we will now look at skills that advance psychotherapy outcomes when robust and hinder progress when deficient. Psychotherapy skills can be divided into interpersonal and non-interpersonal.

INTERPERSONAL SKILLS

Discussions and research examining psychotherapist skills often focus on those of an interpersonal nature. Identified skills include communication, collaboration, rapport building, alliance focus, boundary setting, cultural sensitivity, self-disclosure, and responsiveness (Datta-Barua & Hauser, 2018; Glass, 2003; Priebe et al., 2011; Spencer et al., 2019; Sue, 1998). Psychotherapy relies on communication and skills in this regard are essential: if a therapist cannot communicate effectively and process what the client is expressing psychotherapy will falter. Communication skills that have been identified consist of: positive regard and respect, appropriate involvement in decision making, genuineness, psychological focus, attending to countertransference and transference, active listening and reflection, remaining silent and neutral when appropriate, flexibly responding, and identification of emotions (Datta-Barua & Hauser, 2018; Priebe et al., 2011). A key aspect is a balance of listening with an active component (not drifting off), processing the information, and expressions that are meaningful. Communication skills emphasize expressions that help form

DOI: 10.4324/b23346-14

a bond with the client such as through positive regard, respect, sharing in decision making, and emotionally connected. A study of communication skills training programs for psychiatrists was only able to identify 12 studies, and just 2 randomized controlled trials, with the results indicating that psychotherapeutic interviewing skills and empathy showed improvements (Ditton-Phare et al., 2017). Communication skills can be enhanced through experience combined with attention to what works and what does not, keeping in mind various specific skills. For instance, if your remaining silent and neutral with active listening and reflection is creating uncomfortable gaps in communication, then reduce this component and ramp up expressions.

Ultimately, what counts in the therapeutic relationship is that a solid bond forms, and several therapist skills contribute to this occurrence, a pivotal one being rapport building. To optimize rapport a therapist must think of flexibly aligning themselves with the client so that the person feels accepted and not threatened. Imagine a person saying something that is distasteful to most people and incurring a negative response. In this instance, a therapist must act differently by communicating understanding of the client's perspective in a nonjudgmental fashion. It is often at junctures where most people will respond negatively that rapport is most likely to be advanced via understanding. There are many specific skills that contribute to rapport building, foremost collaboration, self-disclosure, boundary setting, and cultural sensitivity. Approaching the relationship as one of collaboration involving shared decision making is important, even when a client is psychotic. In regard to psychotic clients, I lay out different options and combinations, such as medication and cognitively oriented psychotherapy, and we look at the pluses and minuses of the options with an open exploration of their fears. Anecdotally, I can report much more compliance with medication and psychotherapy through this approach. It is often the case that the more "odd" the person is the more used to being rejected they are, and more appreciative of a collaboration. Collaboration fosters shared meaning and understanding between the subjective inner worlds of the client and therapist, that from an inter-subjectivity/relational perspective has been identified as crucial to forming a robust bond (Buirski & Haglund, 2020; Frayn, 1990; Hasson-Ohayon et al., 2016).

It is not only during the active phase of treatment that collaboration counts, but during the initial sessions (Spencer et al., 2019) and with closure (Goode et al., 2017). Spencer et al. (2019) provide theoretical and research support for establishing a collaboration early in treatment, emphasizing various strategies such as involving the client in decision making, recognizing the client's expertise in treatment, and discussing the possibility of therapist mistakes. Focusing on psychotherapy "termination" Goode et al. (2017) indicate that a collaborative approach helps clients take ownership of gains and equalize the therapeutic relationship, and that "termination" can be discussed throughout sessions, not just at the end. As an aside, I suggest terminating the term, termination, as it does not fit with the nature of psychotherapy, and I doubt that a character such as the Terminator in an Arnold Schwarzenegger movie would perform well as a therapist at the start, middle, or "termination" phase. Closure is superior as it has a positive and constructive feel.

Therapist self-disclosure is a sensitive topic and opinions are all over the map so to speak, highlighting why this is a skill: it is not an either/or matter, but instead an issue of when it is appropriate with real power to advance rapport. For instance, I have a female client who was stalked by a man for a while and still experiences negative feelings about this, reactivated by certain people and social circumstances. Listening to her talk about the situation it emerged that she feels very alone in this regard, because people never seem to understand what it is like. I expressed that I once had a female stalker and indicated that it is difficult for people to appreciate what this entails. Immediately, the rapport which was already good ramped up as she felt a strong connection based on the shared experience. In line with the excellent rapport she let out many feelings about the experience she had never shared. Some therapists will comment that I should not have self-disclosed while others will support it, but the important issue from a skill perspective is knowing and feeling when it will work. With some clients, I share what scuba diving is like, difficult not to talk about given my underwater photographs on the walls, and vary the detail related to the client and their needs at the given moment. Where I have found this self-disclosure really helpful in rapport building is with anxious and avoidant clients, who appreciate my explanation that although scuba diving has challenges, by facing the obstacles very rewarding experiences ensue as evident in the photos. Of interest, many people express that they view scuba diving as a claustrophobic experience, giving me a chance to demonstrate how perspectives can be misleading and inhibiting: scuba diving is actually a very open and free experience, and the closest a person will ever come to flying without mechanical assistance to remain off the ground. This explanation helps anxious and avoidant clients learn that maybe how they view situations might not be accurate, and is blocking them from engaging in potentially rewarding experiences. Self-disclosure is then not only fine but also very helpful from a therapeutic perspective, when it is appropriate and ethical (Barnett, 2011).

Boundary setting might seem to counter rapport building but is actually very important when boundary issues arise, because clients need to know what the boundaries are in the relationship. This is not unique given that all our relationships have boundaries, such as not deceiving friends, and when these boundaries are violated shame tends to arise motivating efforts to rectify the transgression. A key ingredient of being a professional therapist is to have reasonable boundaries and communicate this in a non-offensive fashion when there is the possibility of the client violating them. Clients usually respect this approach, and it assists them in regulating their emotions, because it lays out what is possible and what is not. When a therapist is the one violating boundaries there tends to be a guilty until proven guilty response from regulating bodies and colleagues, with no context applied. Glass (2003) and Gutheil and

Gabbard (1998) recommend making a distinction between boundary cross-ings and boundary violations, with crossings a chance to explore the nature of the relationship, potentially advancing outcomes. Both researchers indicate how there is too much rigidity applied to boundary issues, resulting in too defensive behavior on the part of some clinicians and too punitive a focus, without due consideration of context (Glass, 2003; Gutheil & Gabbard, 1998). Behavior can only be understood with a context. For instance, "She killed a man." What does this mean beyond the obvious? In the absence of context, it is impossible to say. The context of, she was attacked by a rapist and defended herself, is much different than that of, a man she was dating angered her and she stabbed him. Boundary crossings and violations have a context that needs to be applied. For example, a sexual relationship between a client and therapist while always a violation, various with the context. A predatory therapist using the relationship to take advantage of people, is much different than a depressed therapist who just lost his partner engaging in a relationship with a seductive personality disordered client. In the first instance, punitive measures are criti-cal with ejection and termination of the therapist's license (an appropriate use of the term termination), and in the second, therapeutic measures and training might be the solution.

Pertaining to context in the most extreme instance of boundary violations, sexual, McNulty et al. (2013) interviewed three therapists who had engaged in sexual relationships with a client, finding that the following themes applied: therapists' efforts to neutralize power imbalances by minimizing the clients' mental health problems, stressing the conventionality of the relationship and not testing the appropriateness with colleagues or supervisors, and shifting identity of the therapist between hero, victim, and perpetrator. Adding to the context of sexual violations, Norris et al. (2003) indicate that therapist risk factors include: their own life crises, a tendency to idealize a special client, ina-bility to set limits, and denial about the possibility of boundary issues. These diverse themes reinforce the notion that there is a context that is important for therapists to appreciate, hopefully before a violation occurs. Adhering to the role of professional therapist is helpful as roles do have power and provide a sense of the appropriate context. Discussions with colleagues or supervisors about clients that seem to trigger feelings that might lead to boundary vio-lations is strongly recommended, and these consulted individuals do need to apply understanding and assistance. In regard to less severe boundary issues, an interesting contextual issue is small rural communities as discussed by Crowden (2008), who emphasizes dual relationships that are unavoidable, such as your client being the only physiotherapist in town. He recommends that non-exploitive relationships involve professional integrity when there is a potential or actual boundary crossing, which aligns with the notion of adopt-ing and maintaining a professional therapist role even when out of the office. One of the reasons why psychotherapists tend to be clustered in cities and few practice in rural settings, is that the anonymity of cities reduces the stress of dual relationships and boundary issues, but this has the unfortunate consequence of people with mental health needs being out of luck, or having to travel to a city.

Cultural sensitivity is another aspect of rapport building that plays a significant role. In this regard culture is best understood in a broader context than ethnic status, inclusive of sexual orientation, gender, and other "cultural" aspects. While it might be easiest to build rapport with clients that match with your own characteristics, this is not realistic in a world with so much migration and diversity. Empathy and understanding the perspective of clients, as well as learning through experience in therapy and outside of therapy, listening to clients, and reading relevant material comes in handy. Of great significance, humans share many psychotherapy relevant features, such as primary and secondary emotions, psychological regulation capacities, psychological defense mechanism, human specific cognition, and many more. As a humorous contrast, imagine providing psychotherapy to sharks, giraffes, lions, birds, snakes, and dogs. I have found that human similarities are greater than differences, assisting in understanding the experiences and perspectives of other people. Of relevance, some clients will defensively apply differences such as, "You cannot understand what I am going through since you have not experienced severe depression." An empathic and psychologically minded therapist does not have to experience a problem personally to feel and understand the perspective of a client. Likewise, a therapist does not have to be of the same ethnic group, sexual orientation, or gender to work with the client. When defensive expressions of differences occur, it is best for therapists to address how the client might be applying this approach to distance themselves, and express that therapists can appreciate diverse client experiences.

When a therapist is unable to work effectively with cultural differences progress in therapy will be limited. Anderson et al. (2019) conducted an online survey of clients' experiences with psychotherapy, finding that premature "termination" of therapy was more likely with therapists perceived to be low in cultural competence. Vasquez (2007) approaches the matter from a perspective of unintentional biases that interfere with the therapeutic alliance and foster premature dropout from therapy. It is important for therapists to be open about and address these unintentional biases as they set the stage for psychotherapy to fail, and as biases they require reappraisal. Sue (1998) suggests that cognitive match needs to be considered, and that cultural compatibility issues can be overcome by therapists "scientific mindedness," dynamic skills, and culture-specific expertise. On a positive note, broader cultural differences are a chance for the therapist to learn and grow in competency. Of interest and relevance, too great a focus on culture can actually obscure the individual, with the client being seen as a culture and not an individual resulting in an inadequate understanding, despite the cultural sensitivity (Dyche & Zayas, 1995).

Appropriate responsiveness is a skill that contributes to rapport, while also optimizing the application of various therapeutic influences. Hatcher (2015) indicates how this skill yokes to capacities, including empathy and executive functions, organizing and guiding other specific capacities. It refers to how a therapist has to feel, probably more than reason, when, how, and to what extent it is appropriate to respond to clients and apply therapeutic techniques. To a large extent, this capacity is based on what makes a person suitable for a career as a psychotherapist, including solid empathy and psychological mindedness, and advances with experience providing a real "feel" for working with client issues. Although the feel is crucial, inexperienced therapists might have to apply reasoning and utilize executive functions and knowledge to decide on how appropriate a response, such as a transference interpretation or empathic statement, is at the given juncture. This process will become more automatic with experience and learning what is appropriate and what is not based on clients' reactions to your responses.

Although interpersonal psychotherapy skills certainly appear crucial for the success of psychotherapy, it is important to examine the impact of such skills on the process and outcome of therapy. A systematic literature review by Lingiardi et al. (2018), examining the impact of therapist factors spanned 1987 to 2017 identifying 30 relevant studies, with therapists' interpersonal skills and functioning demonstrating the strongest effect on treatment outcome. In a quite rare longitudinal study, Schottke et al. (2017) applied both observer and expert ratings of skills to postgraduate psychotherapy trainees over a five-year stretch, utilizing the Therapy-Related Interpersonal Behaviors (TRIB) scales. They found that observer-rated, but not expert-rated, interpersonal skills showed superior psychotherapy outcomes over the five-year period. Variables that might have confounded the result including therapist related—gender, theoretical orientation (cognitive behavioral or psychodynamic), amount of supervision, client order within the therapist caseload—and client related—age, gender, number of comorbid diagnoses, global severity, and personality disorder problems—did not reduce the effect of the observer-rated therapist interpersonal skills (Schottke et al., 2017).

A major indicator of psychotherapy success is the dropout rate, given that premature termination by the client typically indicates a poor or highly limited outcome. Roos and Werbart (2013) conducted a literature review of dropout from individual psychotherapy, identifying 44 studies between 2000 and 2011. Rates varied widely but the weighted average was 35%, which is actually quite incredible in and of itself, and an indicator that psychotherapy frequently does not progress well (Roos & Werbart, 2013). Most studies did not address therapist, relationship, or process factors, but those that did revealed that therapist skills, experience, and training, together with practical and emotional support, client dissatisfaction, quality of the therapeutic alliance, and pre-therapy preparation, had the greatest impact. The researchers recommend that to reduce dropout rates, thereby improving psychotherapy outcomes, enhanced therapist skills are required and many of these are interpersonal in nature (Roos & Werbart, 2013). Luborsky et al. (2006) in reviewing the caseloads of 22 therapists found that independent of patient background and severity of condition, success rates varied related to efficacy of the therapist with interpersonal skills prominent. In a so-called conceptual review, Priebe et al. (2019) indicate that psychiatric (and not just therapy) skills such as communication, focus on initial contact, empathy, framing of treatments, and decision making, have a greater impact on process (therapeutic relationship, client satisfaction, and adherence) than on more objective outcomes measures such as symptoms and relapse. Of course, if the process goes well, outcomes will likely be better and client satisfaction can be viewed as an outcome. These studies support the position that therapist interpersonal skills do impact on the success of psychotherapy.

Summarizing therapist interpersonal skills: communication, rapport building (collaboration, self-disclosure, boundary setting, and cultural sensitivity), and appropriate responsiveness, stand out as being essential. Conceptual, practical, and research analysis, reveal that when these therapist skills are impaired progress in psychotherapy will be very limited. The incredible 35% dropout rate from psychotherapy is influenced by therapist interpersonal skills (Roos & Werbart, 2013), and hence it is important to address them. Fortunately, interpersonal skills can all be advanced by attention to them and experience in providing psychotherapy.

NON-INTERPERSONAL SKILLS

Therapist skills that are not directly interpersonal are typically not emphasized as much as interpersonal ones, but they have a profound impact on psychotherapy progress. These non-interpersonal skills include techniques, organization, and self-care. Regarding techniques, there are a wide range some very specific to a form of psychotherapy, and others that are more general. Techniques specific to a type of psychotherapy are usually learned during training and practiced with repetition, and are the only non-interpersonal skills that receive significant and ongoing attention. More general ones are where greater variability occurs. Techniques of this nature include: exploration, reflection, interpretations, problem solving, applying related past psychotherapy successes and failures, affect focus, facilitating the expression of affect, and attending to the client's experience (Ackerman & Hilsenroth, 2003). At face value, it is evident that robust general skills will enhance progress in psychotherapy. Exploration assists both the therapist and client in understanding what brings the person into therapy. Reflection furthers this understanding and targets major issues. Interpretations express the products of reflection. Problem solving provides solutions fostering hope. Applying related past psychotherapy successes and failures prevents therapists from repeating mistakes, and maximizes strategies that have worked in the given circumstance. Focusing on affect is important due to how relevant emotions are in problems that bring people to therapy. Facilitating the expression of affect fosters resolution of emotional problems. Attending to the client's experience assists with the therapeutic alliance and understanding what the person is perceiving. Therapists need to consider each of these and do a self-analysis regarding how well they perform on each. When limitations are noted, the best strategy is to consciously focus on the general technique during sessions and practice applying it. Each of the general strategies is well within the capacity of therapists, and so can be improved through practice. Deliberate practice of skills does contribute to the development of highly effective therapists (Chow et al., 2015).

Organizational skills are like software programs that operate in the background enabling the computer to function, including the seamless operation of programs that interface with users. Much like background software they are typically not focused on despite how crucial they are to the success of a psychotherapy practice. During my days of training I cannot recall any mention of organizational skills at all. Fortunately for my practice, I have good organizational skills so it came naturally, but I can only imagine how challenging it is for therapists lacking these skills. Organizational skills are numerous and broad varying with the nature of a therapist's practice but include: office setup, scheduling, contracting with clients regarding various issues, securing payments, referral sources, record keeping, contact and access, and coverage of practice when away. These are only the ones that come to mind and therapists are likely to add several more. Office setup is important as this is what the client experiences right from the start. It involves the layout of the actual office including the waiting room and décor (covered in the Personality Factors chapter). Scheduling is obviously highly relevant and unless a therapist is practicing a scripted form of psychotherapy, such as 12 weekly sessions, there are considerations such as how often a client is to be seen and followed up, which does take some thought. Providing both psychotherapy and medication, I have clients who are seen once a week, once every two, three, four weeks, every two, three, four, five, and six months depending on their needs. This scheduling does take some organization. Then there is the matter of what time of day to see a given client. Some people are not good in the morning so I schedule them in the afternoon, unless they are returning to work after being on disability and have to relearn waking on time; there is nothing like a missed session payment to motivate the client to stop watching shows until the early morning and then sleep in!

Contracting with clients is very important because it clearly lays out expectations, and can be invaluable in the event of a complaint to a regulating body or lawsuit. I contract over attendance and the cost of missed sessions, payment of non-insured services, and other issues that are relevant to only some clients, such as after-hours coverage for personality disorder individuals. Some therapists do not get the person to sign and date but this can be problematic, as in the legal world if it is not papered, so to speak, it is not valid. I have had clients cancel a session late and when I present the charge they say they never heard of this. At this point I pass them the signed and dated agreement. Even though it takes some organization, effort, and confidence to set up contractual agreements with clients, it helps with expectations and boundaries, and protects the therapist. Securing payments largely follows from contracts with clients as these agreements include how payments are to proceed.

Referral sources are what makes a practice viable and attending to this key matter is recommended. When I started practicing psychiatry and psychotherapy, I contacted and actually met with family doctors known to me to explain my practice and the referral process. This personal touch helped set up solid referral sources and let them know what types of clients will not work out, such as extremely unstable personality disorder clients, at least until they stabilize with group therapy. I tend to be quite broad in regard to the mental health problems I treat, so for me it was more identifying what does not work, but therapists with a more specific focus have to make that clear to prospective referral sources. There is no sense focusing on eating disorders and receiving referrals for psychotic clients. Record keeping is required by all regulating bodies and is critical in the event of a complaint or a lawsuit, but beyond these extreme scenarios, it is important to know what transpired and when with each client, and particularly when asked to fill out an insurance form or when a client returns to your practice after a few years. In the old days, records were strictly on paper, but nowadays they are mostly digital which has introduced a slew of stressors and organizational matters for clinicians that require attention.

How clients contact and access their therapist is highly relevant and ties into self-care, because while clients must have some way of contacting you the options cannot lead to therapist burnout. I do not allow regular email or texting options as this becomes far too wearing, and ensures that clients only try and contact me via my office telephone line if there is a real need. I have seen and heard of far too many social workers and psychotherapists burning out, and either quitting their practice or scaling it back to what I would see as a hobby pursuit, due largely to client contacts at night and on weekends. In the spirit of preventing burnout, time away from work is essential raising the concern of coverage while away. For most of my practice an equally busy psychiatrist with an equal interest in travel swapped coverage with me until he retired. At this point, I had to do some additional organizing, and when unable to find a psychiatrist willing to cover my practice, I drafted an emergency coverage sheet that I give to any client that I am at all concerned about, presenting clear options with contact information in the event of a problem. These personal examples show how much organization goes into running a successful psychotherapy practice to the benefit of clients and self-preservation. Like the background software in computers, organization skills keep the practice humming along.

Therapist self-care is presented last but definitely not least! It is like the child and oxygen mask airplane scenario: if the parent focuses too much on the child they pass out and then both suffer or die. Likewise, if a therapist focuses too much on clients and not enough on their own wellbeing they suffer, burnout, and fade from practice to the detriment of both their clients and themselves. I often say that being a martyr is only good for one episode of a show, and since a psychotherapy practice runs over many episodes, being a martyr does not work at all, end of discussion! I present this with some obvious emphasis because working with people is always a stress, and even more when dealing with problems as therapists do; clients do not present saying that everything is great in their life and they want 20 sessions to discuss this. Self-care is arguably the most important psychotherapy skill when considering what makes for a successful busy practice over many years. Some of the self-care aspects relate to organization as with client contact and access, and coverage while away, and by organizing these aspects of your practice with self-care in mind, you will set yourself up for the long run. Another important aspect of self-care is having positive activities fostering dissociative absorption. I believe that my activities including research and writing, skiing, scuba diving and underwater photography, hiking, kayaking, guitar playing, and others have kept my emotional battery charged ongoing. Likewise, a solid social life helps enormously. Trips are also important as they provide an opportunity to engage in hobby pursuits, mental relaxation (psychotherapists rarely need physical relaxation), activity physical and otherwise, and novel experiences that interestingly enough can increase cultural awareness, feeding back on interpersonal therapy skills. Receiving psychotherapy is another ingredient of self-care, but if the other aspects are attended to, then there will be a reduced likelihood of mental health issues requiring psychotherapy. Some forms of psychotherapy, such as psychoanalysis, do require prospective practitioners to engage in therapy during their training, hopefully helping to manage therapist issues that might impede psychotherapy progression. DO NOT neglect self-care if you wish to help clients and maintain your wellbeing over many years!

SUMMARY NOTE

Therapist skills are critical when it comes to helping clients and running a successful psychotherapy practice. Although some skills are more complex and require quite a bit of effort to master, skills are typically easier to improve upon than personality factors making them an ideal focus. Interpersonal skills consist of communication, collaboration, rapport building, alliance focus, boundary setting, cultural sensitivity, self-disclosure, and appropriate responsiveness. Collaboration, self-disclosure, boundary setting, and cultural sensitivity each contribute to rapport building. Non-interpersonal skills consist of specific and general techniques, organization, and self-care. Therapists possessing solid interpersonal and non-interpersonal skills have superior outcomes including lower dropout rates, whereas limited skills greatly impede the progress of psychotherapy. Hence, a focus on the skills presented is strongly recommended for all therapists.

REFERENCES

Ackerman, S. J., & Hilsenroth, M. J. (2003). A review of therapist characteristics and techniques positively impacting on the therapeutic alliance. *Clinical Psychology Review*, *23*(1), 1–33.

Anderson, K. N., Bautista, C. L., & Hope, D. A. (2019). Therapeutic alliance, cultural competence and minority status in premature termination of psychotherapy. *American Journal of Orthopsychiatry*, *89*(1), 104–114.

Barnett, J. E. (2011). Psychotherapist self-disclosure: Ethical and clinical considerations. *Psychotherapy (Chic)*, *48*(4), 315–321.

Buirski, P., & Haglund, P. (2020). *Making sense together: The intersubjective approach to psychotherapy* (2nd ed.). Rowman & Littlefield.

Chow, D. L., Miller, S. D., Seidel, J. A., Kane, R. T., Thornton, J. A., & Andrews, W. P. (2015). The role of deliberate practice in the development of highly effective psychotherapists. *Psychotherapy*, *52*(3), 337–345.

Crowden, A. (2008). Professional boundaries and the ethics of dual and multiple overlapping relationships in psychotherapy. *Monash Bioethics Review*, *27*(4), 10–27.

Datta-Barua, I., & Hauser, J. (2018). Four communication skills from psychiatry useful in palliative care and how to teach them. *AMA Journal of Ethics*, *20*(8), E717–723.

Ditton-Phare, P., Loughland, C., Duvivier, R., & Kelly, B. (2017). Communication skills in the training of psychiatrists: A systematic review of current approaches. *Australian and New Zealand Journal of Psychiatry*, *51*(7), 675–692.

Dyche, L., & Zayas, L. H. (1995). The value of curiosity and naivete for the cross-cultural psychotherapist. *Family Process*, *34*(4), 389–399.

Frayn, D. H. (1990). Intersubjective processes in psychotherapy. *The Canadian Journal of Psychiatry*. https://doi.org/10.1177/070674379003500513

Glass, L. L. (2003). The gray areas of boundary crossings and violations. *American Journal of Psychotherapy*, *57*(4), 429–444.

Goode, J., Park, J., Parkin, S., Tompkins, K. A., & Swift, J. K. (2017). A collaborative approach to psychotherapy termination. *Psychotherapy (Chic)*, *54*(1), 10–14.

Gutheil, T. G., & Gabbard, G. O. (1998). Misuses and misunderstandings of boundary theory in clinical and regulatory settings. *American Journal of Psychiatry*, *155*(3), 409–414.

Hasson-Ohayon, I., Kravetz, S., & Lysaker, P. H. (2016). The special challenge of psychotherapy with persons with psychosis: Intersubjective metacognitive model of agreement and shared meaning. *Clinical Psychology & Psychotherapy*. https://doi.org/10.1002/cpp.2012

Hatcher, R. L. (2015). Interpersonal competencies: Responsiveness, technique, and training in psychotherapy. *American Psychologist*, *70*(8), 747–757.

Lingiardi, V., Muzi, L., Tanzilli, A., & Carone, N. (2018). Do therapists' subjective variables impact on psychodynamic psychotherapy outcomes? A systematic literature review. *Clinical Psychology and Psychotherapy*, *25*(1), 85–101.

Luborsky, L., McLellan, A. T., Diguer, L., Woody, G., & Seligman, D. A. (2006). The psychotherapist matters: Comparison of outcomes across twenty-two therapists and seven patient samples. *Clinical Psychology Science and Practice*. https://doi.org/10.1111/j.1468-2850.1997.tb00099.x

McNulty, N., Ogden, J., & Warren, F. (2013). 'Neutralizing the patient': Therapists' accounts of sexual boundary violations. *Clinical Psychology and Psychotherapy*, *20*(3), 189–199.

Norris, D. M., Gutheil, T. G., & Strasburger, L. H. (2003). This couldn't happen to me: Boundary problems and sexual misconduct in the psychotherapy relationship. *Psychiatric Service*, *54*(4), 517–522.

Priebe, S., Conneely, M., McCabe, R., & Bird, V. (2019). What can clinicians do to improve outcomes across psychiatric treatments: A conceptual review of non-specific components. *Epidemiology Psychiatric Sciences.* https://doi.org/10.1017/s2045796019000428

Priebe, S., Dimic, S., Wildgrube, C., Jankovic, J., Cushing, A., & McCabe, R. (2011). Good communication in psychiatry—A conceptual review. *European Psychiatry, 26*(7), 403–407.

Roos, J., & Werbart, A. (2013). Therapist and relationship factors influencing dropout from individual psychotherapy: A literature review. *Psychotherapy Research, 23*(4), 394–418.

Schottke, H., Fluckiger, C., Goldberg, S. B., Eversmann, J., & Lange, J. (2017). Predicting psychotherapy outcome based on therapist interpersonal skills: A five-year longitudinal study of therapist assessment protocol. *Psychotherapy Research, 27*(6), 642–652.

Spencer, J., Goode, J., Penix, E. A., Trusty, W., & Swift, J. K. (2019). Developing a collaborative relationship with clients during the initial sessions of psychotherapy. *Psychotherapy (Chic), 56*(1), 7–10.

Sue, S. (1998). In search of cultural competence in psychotherapy and counseling. *American Psychologist, 53*(4), 440–448.

Vasquez, M. J. (2007). Cultural difference and the therapeutic alliance: An evidence-based analysis. *American Psychologist, 62*(8), 875–885.

Section III

Interactive Influences

Chapter 13

THERAPEUTIC ALLIANCE

Psychotherapy occurs in a social context with a client and therapist, and so interactive influences are inevitable, the most impactful being the therapeutic alliance, referring to the bond, connection, attachment between the two parties as a key non-specific psychotherapy factor. Ultimately, it is the importance of social connectedness as a state and process for mental health that gives human relationships such power (see the Impaired States and Processes for Mental Health chapter). Even though the alliance between the client and therapist is focused on, any very tight and constructive social alliance has a positive effect on mental health. However, in psychotherapy the bond is pivotal for other therapeutic relationship components to unfold, including trust, openness, caring, support, degree of engagement, positive regard and affirmation, collaboration, overcoming any cultural differences, and agreement over direction (Daniels & Wearden, 2011; Tschacher et al., 2014; Yager & Feinstein, 2017). There is a mutually reinforcing aspect between the therapeutic alliance and these additional relationship factors: the alliance fosters these components and when they are solid the alliance is strengthened. An additional interactive influence occurs with the therapeutic alliance advancing symptom improvement, which in turn enhances the alliance (Falkenstrom et al., 2013). Consistent with the notion of "alliance" both parties play a role. Clients must be willing to make an emotional connection to a therapist and the therapist needs to synch up with the client's emotional experience, the latter dependent on the therapist having a solid empathic ability (see the Emotional Factors chapter).

Considering the significance of the therapeutic alliance, it is understandable that the concept arose in the early days of psychotherapy, with Freud mentioning that the personal emotional relationship between the doctor and patient is stronger than the whole cathartic process (Freud, 1961). Analysts that followed built on the concept, with Zetzel (1956) referring to therapeutic alliance as the healthy part of the client's ego linking up with the analyst to accomplish therapeutic tasks. Carl Rogers (1957, 1986) identified therapist and client influences on the therapeutic relationship: therapist consisting of empathy, congruence (genuineness), and unconditional positive regard, and client involving psychological contact, congruence (alignment of self-image and actual experience),

DOI: 10.4324/b23346-16

and perceptions of the therapist's qualities. Relevant to the therapeutic alliance is the intersubjectivity/relational perspective, emphasizing the shared meaning between the subjective inner worlds of the client and therapist (Buirski & Haglund, 2020). The emergence of this shared meaning contributes substantially to the bond between the client and therapist, and hence the development of a solid therapeutic alliance, which in turn fosters further mutual understanding (Buirski & Haglund, 2020; Frayn, 1990; Hasson-Ohayon et al., 2016).

As transpires with seemingly every concept, clinicians and researchers have created their own unique versions and subtypes of the therapeutic alliance. Greenson (1965) distinguished the working alliance involving the client's capacity to join with the analyst to accomplish tasks, and the therapeutic alliance referring to the personal bond. Luborsky (1976) proposed Type 1 and Type 2 alliances: Type 1 the first phase with the client's belief in the therapist as a source of help, and Type 2 the client's investment in the therapeutic process. Bordin (1994) reframed the therapeutic alliance as a working alliance. In keeping with these distinctions, the therapeutic alliance has been viewed and defined in various ways: independent elements prioritized or synergistic, a stable or changing construct, and a perspective issue varying with who is viewing it such as client, therapist, or observer (Fluckiger et al., 2018). Although there are undoubtedly various aspects to the therapeutic alliance that can be debated at a conceptual level, there is a pure and straightforward feel, motivating mutual commitment to therapy when positive and demotivating commitment when poor. To help understand the therapeutic alliance and the interactive aspect, we will now take a look at what contributes to a solid therapeutic relationship, followed by outcome evidence, and then case examples demonstrating how therapeutic interactions can play out.

FORGING A THERAPEUTIC ALLIANCE

As with relationships outside of a psychotherapy context many factors play a role in the formation of a solid bond, with some the same for client and therapist and others differing. A key example of therapist-based is empathy. In the Emotional Factors chapter, we looked at how empathy is really emotional in nature, enabling the therapist to feel the emotions and understand the emotional perspective of the client. When a client perceives the therapist's empathy, the person is much more likely to trust the therapist and express feelings and thoughts, that if responded appropriately to by the therapist further foster the therapeutic alliance. Hence, it is really very interactive. A review of 53 studies by Nienhuis et al. (2018) found that the therapeutic alliance was significantly related to client perceptions of therapist empathy, highlighting the interaction between empathy on the part of the therapist and client perceptions.

Research has examined what contributes to the therapeutic alliance beyond empathy. Given that the alliance is about bonding and attachment, it follows that the attachment styles of both the client and therapist have an influence.

Secure attachment arises from supportive, sensitive, and responsive parenting (Bee & Boyd, 2004). Insecure attachment transpires when caregivers are non-responsive, inconsistent, and fail to support a child producing doubts about oneself and others (Atwool, 2006). Secure attachment facilitates social bonding, such as occurs in the therapeutic relationship. Not surprisingly, research does show that for both clients and therapists secure attachment fosters a healthy therapeutic alliance (Diener & Monroe, 2011; Slade & Holmes, 2019; Smith et al., 2010; Steel et al., 2018). Applying a systematic review, Smith et al. (2010) discovered that despite inconsistencies in terms of measurement and conceptualization of attachment and alliance, clients who rate themselves as having a more secure attachment pattern rate the therapeutic alliance as stronger. A meta-analysis of 17 psychotherapy studies by Diener and Monroe (2011) found that client attachment security was associated with stronger therapeutic alliances, whereas attachment insecurity linked to weaker therapeutic alliances. Steel et al. (2018) performed a systematic review examining therapist attachment with 19 relevant studies, concluding that therapist attachment impacts the therapeutic alliance in terms of relationship quality based on client-rated evaluations, therapist negative countertransference, empathy, and problems in therapy. Insecure attachment led to a lower quality therapeutic relationship while secure attachment resulted in a higher quality one (Steel et al., 2018). Reviewing attachment and psychotherapy considering the contribution of both the client and therapist, Slade and Holmes (2019) found that client insecure attachment contributes to therapy ruptures and in-session problems, while therapist insecure attachment impacts on the success of psychotherapy.

Insecure attachment involves distrust and doubts about other people derived from early life caregiver experiences, clearly impacting on a person's willingness and even capacity to form social bonds. Secure attachment, on the other hand, sets the stage for bonding as a natural default pattern. Interactions transpire, as when client and therapist both have secure attachment patterns a robust relationship is more likely to form, but if one, or worse, both have insecure attachment patterns, then the therapeutic alliance is challenged from the start. When insecure attachment exists, the client and/or therapist have to revisit their early life relationships with caregivers and see how the interaction favored distrust. A crucial learning component consists of realizing that although in the early years of life a person does not have a choice of who to associate with nor control over relationships, adulthood does enable choice and control, with this realization being very empowering. Practicing choice and control (or at least influence) in current relationships provides a powerful corrective emotional experience.

Communication is another contributor to the therapeutic alliance, with research focused on therapist communication. Kadur et al. (2020) conducted a systematic review of therapist communication and the impact on the therapeutic alliance and outcomes. The 10 articles reviewed revealed that supportive and exploratory statements, and addressing the therapeutic relationship, were beneficial, whereas controlling and challenging statements weakened the alliance and outcomes (Kadur et al., 2020). In another systematic review, Pinto et al. (2012) found that in therapeutic relationships the alliance is strengthened by listening to clients, and asking questions demonstrating sensitivity to the client's emotional needs, obviously yoking to empathy. Focusing on communication in medicine and psychiatry, Cruz and Pincus (2002) reviewed 25 studies in medicine and 34 in psychiatry covering 1950–2001. This comprehensive review showed that good communication increases patient satisfaction, adherence to treatment recommendations, outcomes, and willingness to file malpractice claims (Cruz & Pincus, 2002). It is important to note that although the psychotherapy alliance is mostly the focus of research, every client and treatment provider relationship benefits from a solid therapeutic alliance!

Client communication also plays a significant role because if a person does not express emotional and other information, it is challenging for the therapist to bond to the person. Every psychotherapist has had the experience of clients who do not voluntarily speak, and when open ended questions are tried they respond with a curtailed sentence and no more. In these instances, therapy usually does not progress beyond the assessment or initial sessions, partly due to an alliance failing to form. Of note, when it comes to mental health issues, therapists rely on verbal information from the client, while with general medicine there is the assistance of lab tests and radiological investigations. Psychotherapy is very communication oriented and both client and therapist play a role. In the case of the psychotherapist, if communication problems exist as an ongoing issue, as opposed to just with a particularly client, then communication skills training can assist. For clients, I have found that involvement with Toastmasters helps with communication beyond presentations, as the person learns clear and assertive expression.

Various therapist characteristics beyond attachment and communication have been linked to a solid therapeutic alliance. A review by Timulak and Keogh (2017) identified willingness to seek client perspectives, openness to hearing what the client has to say, non-defensiveness in the face of negative feedback, and ability to modulate actions to achieve better collaboration. In another review, Ackerman and Hilsenroth (2003) cite personal attributes— flexible, honest, respectful, trustworthy, confident, warm, interested, and open—and techniques—exploration, reflection, noting past therapy successes and setbacks, accurate interpretation, facilitating the expression of affect, and attending to the client's experience—as fostering a good therapeutic alliance. In an earlier review of the literature, Ackerman and Hilsenroth (2001) found that therapist's personal attributes including being rigid, uncertain, critical, distant, tense, and distracted, contribute negatively to the therapeutic alliance. Therapist techniques, such as over structuring the therapy session, inappropriate self-disclosure, unyielding use of transference interpretations, and application of excessive silence, also contribute to a poor therapeutic alliance (Ackerman & Hilsenroth, 2001). In the Skills Factors chapter, we looked at how appropriate responsiveness and rapport building are very important, with collaboration, self-disclosure, boundary setting, and cultural sensitivity contributing to the latter capacity. Even very straightforward and simple therapist interventions can build rapport and advance the therapeutic alliance: Duff and Bedi (2010) conducted a regression analysis of 15 behaviors that might be linked to a solid therapeutic alliance, discovering that making encouraging statements, positive comments about the client, and greeting the client with a smile accounted for 62% of alliance scores! By focusing on the various characteristics associated with a solid therapeutic alliance and trying to improve them, a therapist can optimize the relationship.

A robust therapeutic alliance then relies on the client and therapist. Secure attachment and communication apply to both the client and therapist. Empathy, rapport building, and appropriate responsiveness stand out as crucial for the therapist, but it is easy to imagine how clients with greater capacities in regard to these key therapist factors will forge a stronger alliance. Several other therapist factors play a role, many consisting of skills that can be improved upon by the therapist consciously focusing on them in sessions and practicing their application. Even personality factors relevant to the therapeutic alliance (see the Personality Factors chapter), such as openness and agreeableness, can be advanced simply by experience providing therapy as this enhances these traits (Grunberger & Laireiter, 2013), and also by adopting the role of professional therapist and expressing openness and agreeableness as part of this role. The focus on the therapeutic alliance is based on the assumption that it influences the success of psychotherapy, necessitating a look at the evidence.

OUTCOME EVIDENCE

The therapeutic alliance is one of the most researched psychotherapy concepts, and outcome evidence is a focus. A meta-analysis of 11 studies involving 1,301 participants by Sharf et al. (2010) focused on the dropout rate, finding that clients who experienced a weaker therapeutic alliance were significantly more likely to dropout of therapy. Moderating variables including lower client education, shorter treatment length, and outpatient psychotherapy, were associated with higher dropout rates (Sharf et al., 2010). Samstag et al. (1998) discovered that when both the client and therapist rated the alliance as problematic dropout rates were higher. In their review study reported earlier, Roos and Werbart (2013) found that the quality of the therapeutic alliance contributes to the staggering 35% dropout rate from psychotherapy. Applying a meta-analysis of data from 79 studies, Martin et al. (2000) noted a moderate but consistent relationship between the therapeutic alliance and outcome. Of interest, various moderator variables including the type of outcome measure, type of outcome rater, type of alliance rater, timing of alliance assessment, type of treatment provided, and publication status did not have any influence on the relationship between the therapeutic alliance and outcome of therapy (Martin et al., 2000).

Outcome research has looked at various mental health problems and interventions, with the therapeutic alliance consistently linked to superior outcomes.

A National Institute of Mental Health study involving 225 clients with depression, evaluated those receiving interpersonal therapy, cognitive-behavioral therapy, an antidepressant, or a placebo medication (Krupnick et al., 1996). Clinician raters scored videotaped sessions for the therapeutic alliance, and outcome was rated by both clients and evaluators. The quality of the therapeutic alliance had a significant effect on clinical outcome in all conditions, including the placebo medication (Krupnick et al., 1996)! Likewise focusing on depression treatment, Klein et al. (2003) applied cognitive behavioral analysis system of psychotherapy to 367 participants, finding that an early alliance significantly predicted improvement in depressive symptoms. Examining self-harm and suicidal behavior, Dunster-Page et al. (2017) reviewed 12 studies discovering that patient-rated alliance had the strongest impact on self-harm behaviors. Plakun (2001) suggests that the therapeutic alliance represents an edge or boundary across which the survival of the client (and therapy) can be negotiated, and as such, attention to the alliance by the therapist is critical when it comes to managing suicidal behavior. Trauma is a common focus in psychotherapy, and quite often involves personality disorder pathology and self-harm. Ellis et al. (2018) performed a systematic review of 19 studies between 1980 and 2015, discovering that the vast majority showed the therapeutic alliance to be predictive of, or associated with, a reduction in trauma symptoms.

Psychosis and schizophrenic spectrum disorders constitute extreme mental illness manifestation. Browne et al. (2019) reviewed 84 studies examining the relationship between the therapeutic alliance and outcomes when these conditions were involved. Better client ratings of the alliance were associated with superior insight, medication adherence, social support, and recovery variables, while therapist ratings linked to medication adherence, less severe symptoms, and recovery variables. Likewise focusing on psychotic illnesses, Shattock et al. (2018) conducted a systematic review of 26 studies, finding that a better alliance predicted overall psychotic symptom outcomes. Poorer insight and sexual abuse contributed to worse client-rated alliance, whereas negative symptoms were associated with worse therapist-rated alliance (Shattock et al., 2018).

Eating disorders can be challenging to treat and the therapeutic alliance plays a role in outcomes. Graves et al. (2017) performed a meta-analysis of 20 studies, discovering small to medium effect sizes for the therapeutic alliance on symptom reduction, and that early symptom improvement positively influenced the therapeutic alliance. Young people suffer from eating disorders and other problems, and conceivably the therapeutic alliance might have a different impact on outcomes with this population than it does for adults. Looking into this possibility, Murphy and Hutton (2018) did a systematic review and meta-analysis of adolescents receiving treatment for diverse problems, finding that the relationship between therapeutic alliance and outcome was higher than previously reported. Green (2006) investigated the therapeutic alliance in children with mental health issues, noting that it applies as with older clients, and appears to have a more significant influence on outcomes when externalizing disorders are present. This relationship between externalizing behavior and the therapeutic alliance was repeated in a study by Hogue et al. (2006), who discovered that in family therapy, but not cognitive behavioral therapy, adolescents treated for substance abuse who demonstrated an improved therapeutic alliance, experienced a reduction in externalizing behaviors compared to those for whom the therapeutic alliance declined.

Psychotherapy is mostly face to face, but technological modes of delivery including videoconferencing, Internet, email, and telephone are becoming increasingly common. The question arises: Does the therapeutic alliance suffer as a result? Reviewing eight studies focusing on the treatment of depression, Wehmann et al. (2020) did not find any differences between client ratings of the alliance when technology was applied compared to in-person sessions. Examining six studies of Internet-delivered cognitive behavioral therapy for depression and anxiety, Pihlaja et al. (2017) noted a high client-therapist alliance, and the three most recent studies found that the alliance was positively associated with outcome. In a narrative review, Berger (2017) notes that independent of communication modalities, diagnostic groups, and amount of contact between clients and therapists, client-rated alliance is high and roughly comparable to that with in-person sessions. Hence, in response to the question posed, technology based modes of psychotherapy delivery do not seem to impede the therapeutic alliance, aligning with how all forms of social activity seem to work for mental health (Bowins, 2020). Performing a broad review of "telemental health" Lopez et al. (2019) discovered that therapists have more concerns about the alliance than do clients, who seem to adjust better.

To this point, the review has emphasized the relationship between the therapeutic alliance and outcome of therapy. Taking a different perspective on the therapeutic alliance and highlighting how it is not all about outcome, Catty (2004) indicates that it might be best conceptualized as a "vehicle" for treatment assisting in the delivery of other influences, rather than curative in and of itself. Catty (2004) indicates that the focus on outcome is derived from empirical psychotherapy research, due to outcome being quite measurable. Realistically, the therapeutic alliance is likely both a "vehicle" for the application of other psychotherapy relevant factors, as mentioned at the start of the chapter, and an influence on outcome given the potency of high quality relationships and social connectedness for mental health.

CASE EXAMPLES

For a solid therapeutic alliance to form it really does require participation of both the client and therapist, ensuring that interactions are highly relevant. Based on attachment patterns and communication contributing to the alliance, I will provide examples of therapeutic alliance interactions involving these influences. Therapist empathy also weighs in heavily, but as mentioned, a non-empathic therapist is not likely to succeed and remain in the career.

The therapeutic alliance forms readily when both the client and therapist have secure attachment patterns, my therapy with Betty providing an example. She experienced severe depression in her 40s only resolved via behavioral therapy, with medications of very limited benefit. Facilitating her rapid progress was a robust therapeutic alliance with a great deal of trust in what I suggested: she was skeptical of behavioral therapy but expressed that she trusted me and so tried it, adhering to the step-wise strategies we worked out. Bonding and alliance formation came easily for her, as both parents were highly supportive and caring always looking out for her interests. She actually ended up suffering because she trusted people too easily, and was taken advantage of by repair people, some "friends," and also her brother who was a "wheeler and dealer" focused on money. He took advantage of her trust and monopolized money from the estate of their parents. These setbacks, and primarily that involving her brother, triggered the depression. Given that both her and my attachment patterns are secure, the bond formed rapidly and assisted in her working with me to increase her positive activities and distance herself from negativity. She made an impressive improvement in relatively short time.

Communication assisted as Betty expressed herself well, including any fears or reservations, and also very importantly, feelings of embarrassment and "stupidity" for being taken advantage of. Therapy involved self-awareness that she trusts too easily and sets herself up for being manipulated, and relevant to communication, I expressed that if I had negative intentions I could have manipulated her given the implicit trust. She found this statement revealing as she realized that her default pattern is to trust and bond, but select people have used this to manipulate her. We worked on looking for red flags, and conducting a due diligence whenever she stands to lose. With this knowledge and understanding she now carefully scrutinizes any potential relationship opportunity, as well as repair people asking for references, and seeks my feedback if uncertain. This more defensive posture has stopped her from being taken advantage of resulting in no further depression, better self-concept, and stable finances. An interaction transpired given that the bond helped her advance and the solid connection motivated me to invest to the maximum extent in her progress, which in turn increased her commitment to treatment, and so on and so forth. The fast and solid progress was attributable to the robust therapeutic alliance, derived from secure attachment, and good communication, and the mutually reinforcing therapeutic alliance features.

In contrast to the example involving Betty, the therapeutic alliance is challenged when issues with attachment and communication transpire. In her early 50s, Julia presented with depression related to a career issue. A change of manager left her feeling unsupported in her bank job, and progressively critiqued, although she believed she knew her job well and the prior manager was fine with her performance. Julia sensed that her colleagues were losing faith in her, likely derived from how the new manager treated her in team meetings. These feelings of alienation were partly transference related, as her father was largely absent and controlling when around, while her mother provided limited support. She repeated the pattern involving her father by marrying a man who was controlling and aloof. Her attachment pattern based on these early, and also adult, life experiences was predominantly insecure. Despite this attachment pattern, she showed the capacity to bond to supportive people, such as her prior manager, perhaps derived from some support by her mother. Hence, I had the sense that she could bond to me, which would further her progress. What interfered was a conflict between various desires, and strained communication as a result.

Due to the work situation and ensuing depression, she went on insurance disability supported by her family doctor, who then referred her to me. Normally in these scenarios I provide psychotherapy and/or medication as required, the client improves, and returns to work with a plan. Julia though was heavily conflicted between a desire to have a career and avoid the work setting altogether, and also leave her husband or stay, with leaving easier if she did not have a job, as in this scenario she would not have to support him financially. Consequently, she was not always so open about what she was experiencing, and in particular about any improvements, as resolution of symptoms might have paved the way for a return to work. Despite the insecure attachment pattern and conflicts, I continued to sense the potential for a solid bond, and even a positive transference of a supportive and non-controlling male figure, but the complex interaction between her mental health issues, career, disability, and marriage problems interfered. For several months, Julia was in a "limbo state" caught in a difficult scenario where every move had limitations from her perspective. Her situation resolved when the insurance company terminated her support, and with my encouragement she had a lawyer negotiate a severance package with the employer. Her mood gradually improved and she thanked me for the support, and also focus on how the ambivalent state maintained the depression. From this point on she opened up about her feelings, and in particular, those pertaining to her husband and the poor marriage. She strongly feels that she will never be emotionally close to her husband due to the ongoing control he exerts over her and his aloofness, and does see how she has repeated the history with her father, neither relationship feasible to improve. Currently, she is considering leaving the marriage and moving to new location where she will start a more appealing career. The example of Julia demonstrates how even if a client has insecure attachment she or he still has the potential to bond, but this can interact with circumstances to limit communication and block a solid therapeutic alliance until the interfering situation is resolved.

Interactions between attachment patterns and communication can take many interesting forms varying with extraneous factors. Gregory provides a unique example of how despite secure attachment capacity present with both client and therapist, therapy failed related to issues involving communication. A young man in his late 20s, Gregory had a very close relationship with his father, and also his mother but to a lesser extent. His parents divorced when he was very young and he primarily lived with his father. Understandably he was devastated emotionally when his father died suddenly, and this triggered a depressive episode that took a while to recover from. Financially, he was set up very well as his father left all assets including a house to him, enabling Gregory to progress with his writing ambitions. My involvement came a few years later when he discovered that his mood was low again, but not fully depressed as when his father died. Gregory was lost in his career, as despite getting one book published by a small press, he felt blocked with further writings. Given that I am male and write, with both of us having a secure attachment pattern, the potential for a close therapeutic alliance was feasible. Unfortunately, it was scuttled very early related to various circumstances and communication issues.

Initially it felt like a bond was starting to form, with Gregory appreciating my experience writing and my identifying with a young aspiring writer. Then an event occurred that set things back. It was obvious that he had far too much time on his hands, and the saying that the longer one has to do something the longer it takes applied. He procrastinated, sat around, and engaged in very little productive effort. We were starting to work on how if he acquired even a part-time job his writing productivity would ironically advance, given that he would shift into an active mode. After the start time of our next session I received a call from Gregory, with him saying that due to a subway issue he bypassed the station for my office. He thought he could make it and did but just prior to the end of the session. I agreed to have a short session, but warned him that if it repeats there will be a charge. At this point he became angry and expressed that this is wrong as it was a subway problem. During the assessment I expressed to him, as I do with every client, that due to the endless construction in the area and subway delays, clients need to arrive early as I have to charge for missed sessions, and how my office location has many options for relaxing prior to a session. I understand that for very busy clients this will not be realistic at times, but for a young man with more time on his hands than is imaginable, arriving well before the session is very feasible. He expressed that he did not recall that explanation and believed he did what he could. Before I could investigate potential transference issues and/or resolve the disagreement, the COVID-19 pandemic hit and he ended therapy likely related to the conflict. The example of Gregory highlights how the potential for a solid therapeutic bond, derived from both the client and therapist having secure attachment patterns, can falter related to communication.

Even when a client has insecure attachment empathic communication can forge a solid bond, as demonstrated by Dan, a long-term client who I see about once per month now. Dan's early life was very stressful growing up in a small town setting in Eastern Canada, his mother schizophrenic and father probably having bipolar disorder. Making matters worse for Dan, the social environment was all about being macho for boys with sports involvements, which did not interact well with his artistic leanings. Dan was bullied and ostracized, which in combination with very distant parenting ensured an insecure attachment pattern. When he presented for an assessment he was in his early 30s, and expressed that he had tried a couple of therapists but did not feel that it was working. He ventured that there are sexual issues that are difficult to discuss. I expressed that I have heard many things and can assist him. He visibly relaxed at this juncture and explained that he is sexually drawn to children, mostly boys but girls too, but has not acted on these urges. His expressive communication was reciprocated with me expressing what he clearly did not expect: praise that he had not acted on these urges and a follow-up that people have many sexual desires that do not slot into the narrow socially prescribed views, and what really counts is what you do with those urges. That supportive statement led to years of trust and a solid bond, enabling him to freely express his desires, fears, and self-concept issues. Dan felt shame and self-loathing for having these urges, but became more accepting of them when we looked at the distorted world view presented by his parents, and ostracism by his peers. He realized that he did not create these sexual preferences, and was actually acting ethically by ensuring he never acted on them. Several years later he was shocked to hear that his only brother was charged with molesting a step-child, further reinforcing the reality that he did not select his sexual preference, and was actually strong of character for not acting on the urges. We worked on managing his sexual desires, including sublimating the energy into constructive endeavors, which has contributed to a successful arts career. Dan's example reveals that with the right communication and openness on the part of the therapist, a solid therapeutic alliance can form when the client has insecure attachment.

The examples provided illustrate how interactive the therapeutic alliance is. I focused on attachment patterns and communication as they clearly contribute to the alliance between client and therapist. As the example of Gregory reveals therapy can falter even when both parties have a secure attachment pattern, and certainly if communication is strained. Dan's example shows that a person with insecure attachment can forge a very robust therapeutic alliance with the right communication and openness. The potential for a good bond can be disrupted by extraneous influences impacting on communication as with Julia. Then there is the ideal scenario of Betty, whereby both the client and therapist have secure attachment and communication is unimpeded, that leads to really impressive outcomes. Empathy plays a key role in the therapeutic alliance, but the assumption here is that the therapist will most likely be advanced in this regard. If not, then many other interactions can emerge, most not positive for the therapeutic alliance and the outcome of therapy.

SUMMARY NOTE

The notion of a therapeutic alliance as a bond, connection, attachment between client and therapist, has been around since the early days of psychotherapy, and has stood up very well as a non-specific factor. Key contributors include therapist empathy, client and therapist attachment patterns and communication, and therapist characteristics and skills with rapport building and appropriate responsiveness being very important. Supporting the relevance of the therapeutic alliance, research consistently finds a link between a solid therapeutic alliance and psychotherapy outcomes over many different conditions and client ages. The examples provided demonstrate how interactions between attachment patterns and communication can play out, and not always as straightforward as secure attachment for both parties resulting in good outcomes and insecure attachment poor outcomes. The potential for a good therapeutic alliance can be impeded by extraneous factors, and the right communication can overcome a client's insecure attachment. These interactions make psychotherapy both interesting and challenging, which is where therapist skill and empathy really come in.

REFERENCES

Ackerman, S. J., & Hilsenroth, M. J. (2001). A review of therapist characteristics and techniques negatively impacting the therapeutic alliance. *Psychotherapy: Theory, Research, Practice, Training*, *38*(2), 171–185.

Ackerman, S. J., & Hilsenroth, M. J. (2003). A review of therapist characteristics and techniques positively impacting on the therapeutic alliance. *Clinical Psychology Review*, *23*(1), 1–33.

Atwool, N. (2006). Attachment and resilience: Implications for children in care. *Child Care in Practice*, *12*, 315–330.

Bee, H. L., & Boyd, D. (2004). *The developing child* (10th ed.). Allyn & Bacon.

Berger, T. (2017). The therapeutic alliance in internet interventions: A narrative review and suggestions for future research. *Psychotherapy Research*, *27*(5), 511–524.

Bordin, E. S. (1994). Theory and research on the therapeutic working alliance: New directions. In A. O. Horvath & L. S. Greenberg (Eds.), *The working alliance: Theory, research, and practice* (pp. 13–37). Wiley.

Bowins, B. E. (2020). *Activity for mental health*. Academic Press.

Browne, J., Nagendra, A., Kurtz, M., Berry, K., & Penn, D. L. (2019). The relationship between the therapeutic alliance and client variables in individual treatment for schizophrenic spectrum disorders and early psychosis: Narrative review. *Clinical Psychology Review*, *71*, 51–62.

Buirski, P., & Haglund, P. (2020). *Making sense together: The intersubjective approach to psychotherapy* (2nd ed.). Rowman & Littlefield.

Catty, J. (2004). The vehicle of success': Theoretical and empirical perspectives on the therapeutic alliance in psychotherapy and psychiatry. *Psychology and Psychotherapy*, *77*(2), 255–272.

Cruz, M., & Pincus, H. A. (2002). Research on the influence that communication in psychiatric encounters has on treatment. *Psychiatric Service*, *53*(10), 1253–1265.

Daniels, J., & Wearden, A. J. (2011). Socialization to the model: The active component in the therapeutic alliance? A preliminary study. *Behavioural and Cognitive Psychotherapy*, *39*(2), 221–227.

Diener, M. J., & Monroe, J. M. (2011). The relationship between adult attachment and therapeutic alliance in individual psychotherapy: A meta-analytic review. *Psychotherapy*, *48*(3), 237–248.

Duff, C. T., & Bedi, R. P. (2010). Counsellor behaviors that predict therapeutic alliance: From the client's perspective. *Counselling Psychology Quarterly*. https://doi.org/10.1080/09515071003688165

Dunster-Page, C., Haddock, G., Wainwright, L., & Berry, K. (2017). The relationship between therapeutic alliance and patient's suicidal thoughts, self-harming behaviors and suicide attempts: A systematic review. *Journal of Affective Disorders, 223*, 165–174.

Ellis, A. E., Simiola, V., Brown, L., Courtois, C., & Cook, J. M. (2018). The role of evidence-based therapy relationships on treatment outcomes for adults with trauma: A systematic review. *Journal of Trauma and Dissociation, 19*(2), 185–213.

Falkenstrom, F., Granstrom, F., & Holmqvist, R. (2013). Therapeutic alliance predicts symptomatic improvement session by session. *Journal of Counselling Psychology, 60*(3), 317–328.

Fluckiger, C., Del Re, A. C., Wampold, B. E., & Horvath, A. O. (2018). The alliance in adult psychotherapy: A meta-analytic synthesis. *Psychotherapy (Chic), 55*(4), 316–340.

Frayn, D. H. (1990). Intersubjective processes in psychotherapy. *The Canadian Journal of Psychiatry*. https://doi.org/10.1177/070674379003500513

Freud, S. (1961). The future of an illusion, civilization and its discontents, and other works. In J. Starchey (Ed.), *The standard edition of the complete psychological works of Sigmund Freud* (Vol. 21, pp. 5–68). Hogarth. (Original work published 1927.)

Graves, T. A., Tabri, N., Thompson-Brenner, H., Franko, D. L., Eddy, K. T., Bourion-Bedes, S., et al. (2017). A meta-analysis of the relation between therapeutic alliance and treatment outcomes in eating disorders. *International Journal of Eating Disorders, 50*(4), 323–340.

Green, J. (2006). Annotation: The therapeutic alliance—a significant but neglected variable in child mental health treatment studies. *Journal of Child Psychology and Psychiatry, 47*(5), 425–435.

Greenson, R. R. (1965). The working alliance and the transference neurosis. *The Psychoanalytic Quarterly, 34*, 155–181.

Grunberger, T., & Laireiter, A. R. (2013). Between growth and isolation—The influence of therapy on the experience and the personality of therapists. *Psychotherapy and Psychosomatics, 64*(1), 28–34.

Hasson-Ohayon, I., Kravetz, S., & Lysaker, P. H. (2016). The special challenge of psychotherapy with persons with psychosis: Intersubjective metacognitive model of agreement and shared meaning. *Clinical Psychology & Psychotherapy*. https://doi.org/10.1002/cpp.2012

Hogue, A., Dauber, S., Stambaugh, L. F., Cecero, J. J., & Liddle, H. A. (2006). Early therapeutic alliance and treatment outcome in individual and family therapy for adolescent behavior problems. *Journal of Consulting and Clinical Psychology, 74*(1), 121–129.

Kadur, J., Ludemann, J., & Andreas, S. (2020). Effects of the therapist's statements on the patient's outcome and the therapeutic alliance: A systematic review. *Clinical Psychology and Psychotherapy, 27*(2), 168–178.

Klein, D. N., Schwartz, J. E., Santiago, N. J., Vivian, D., Vocisano, C., Castonguay, L. G., et al (2003). Therapeutic alliance in depression treatment: Controlling for prior change and patient characteristics. *Journal of Consulting and Clinical Psychology, 71*(6), 997–1006.

Krupnick, J. L., Sotsky, S. M., Simmens, S., Moyer, J., Elkin, I., Watkins, J., et al. (1996). The role of the therapeutic alliance in psychotherapy and pharmacotherapy outcome: Findings in the National Institute of Mental Health Treatment of Depression Collaborative Research Program. *Journal of Consulting and Clinical Psychology*. https://doi.org/10.1037//0022-006x.64.3.532

Lopez, A., Schwenk, S., Schneck, C. D., Griffin, R. J., & Mishkind, M. C. (2019). Technology-based mental health treatment and the impact on the therapeutic alliance. *Current Psychiatry Reports*. https://doi.org/10.1007/s11920-019-1055-7

Luborsky, L. (1976). Helping alliances in psychotherapy. In J. L. Cleghhorn (Ed.), *Successful psychotherapy* (pp. 92–116). Brunner/Mazel.

Martin, D. J., Garske, J. P., & Davis, M. K. (2000). Relation of the therapeutic alliance with outcome and other variables: A meta-analytic review. *Journal of Consulting and Clinical Psychology*, 68(3), 438–450.

Murphy, R., & Hutton, P. (2018). Practitioner review: Therapist variability, patient-reported therapeutic alliance, and clinical outcomes in adolescents undergoing mental health treatment—A systematic review and meta-analysis. *Journal of Child Psychology and Psychiatry*, 59(1), 5–19.

Nienhuis, J. B., Owen, J., Valentine, J. C., Black, S. W., Halford, T. C., Parazak, S. E., et al. (2018). Therapeutic alliance, empathy, and genuineness in individual adult psychotherapy: A meta-analytic review. *Psychotherapy Research*, 28(4), 593–605.

Pihlaja, S., Sternberg, J. H., Joutsenniemi, K., Mehik, H., Ritola, V., & Joffe, G. (2017). Therapeutic alliance in guided internet therapy programs for depression and anxiety disorders—A systematic review. *Internet Interventions*. https://doi.org/10.1016/j.invent.2017.11.005

Pinto, R. Z., Ferreira, M. L., Oliveira, V. C., Franco, M. R., Adams, R., Maher, P. H., et al. (2012). Patient-centred communication is associated with positive therapeutic alliance: A systematic review. *Journal of Physiotherapy*, 58(2), 77–87.

Plakun, E. M. (2001). Making the alliance and taking the transference in work with suicidal patients. *Journal of Psychotherapy Practice and Research*, 10(4), 269–276.

Rogers, C. R. (1957). The necessary and sufficient conditions of therapeutic personality change. *Journal of Consulting Psychology*, 21(2), 95–103.

Rogers, C. R. (1986). Carl Rogers on the development of the person-centered approach. *Person-Centered Review*, 1(3), 257–259.

Roos, J., & Werbart, A. (2013). Therapist and relationship factors influencing dropout from individual psychotherapy: A literature review. *Psychotherapy Research*, 23(4), 394–418.

Samstag, L. W., Batchelder, S. T., Muran, J. C., Safran, J. D., & Winston, A. (1998). Early identification of treatment failures in short-term psychotherapy: An assessment of therapeutic alliance and interpersonal behavior. *Journal of Psychotherapy Practice and Research*, 7(2), 126–143.

Sharf, J., Primavera, L. H., & Diener, M. J. (2010). Dropout and therapeutic alliance: A meta-analysis of adult individual psychotherapy. *Psychotherapy: Theory, Research, Practice, Training*, 47(4), 637–645.

Shattock, L., Berry, K., Degnan, A., & Edge, D. (2018). Therapeutic alliance in psychological therapy for people with schizophrenia and related psychosis: A systematic review. *Clinical Psychology and Psychotherapy*, 25(1), 60–65.

Slade, A., & Holmes, J. (2019). Attachment and psychotherapy. *Current Opinions in Psychology*, 25, 152–156.

Smith, A. E., Msetfi, R. M., & Golding, L. (2010). Client self-rated adult attachment patterns and the therapeutic alliance: A systematic review. *Clinical Psychology Review*, 30(3), 326–337.

Steel, C., Macdonald, J., & Schroder, T. (2018). A systematic review of the effects of therapists' internalized models of relationships on the quality of the therapeutic relationship. *Journal of Clinical Psychology*, 74(1), 5–42.

Timulak, L., & Keogh, D. (2017). The client's perspective on (experiences of) psychotherapy: A practice friendly review. *Journal of Clinical Psychology*, 73(11), 1156–1567.

Tschacher, W., Junghan, U. M., & Pfammatter, M. (2014). Towards a taxonomy of common factors in psychotherapy—Results from an expert survey. *Clinical Psychology and Psychotherapy*, *21*(1), 82–96.

Wehmann, E., Kohnen, M., Harter, M., & Liebherz, S. (2020). Therapeutic alliance in technology-based interventions for the treatment of depression: Systematic review. *Journal of Medical Internet Research*. https://doi.org/10.2196/17195

Yager, J., & Feinstein, R. E. (2017). Tools for practical psychotherapy: A transtheoretical collection (or interventions which have, at least, worked for us). *Journal of Psychiatric Practice*, *23*(1), 60–77.

Zetzel, E. R. (1956). Current concepts of transference. *The International Journal of Psychoanalysis*, *37*, 369–376.

Chapter 14

INTERACTIONS BETWEEN CLIENT AND THERAPIST INFLUENCES

The various client and therapist influences covered in the first and second sections, respectively, do interact, impacting psychotherapy progress both directly and via the therapeutic alliance. The client influences chapters in the first section consist of: Motivation, Expectations, Personality Disorders, Reinforcement Parameters, Complexity, Resistance and Noncompliance, Impaired States and Processes for Mental Health, and Transference. The therapist influences chapters consist of: Countertransference, Emotional Factors, Personality Factors, and Skill Factors. Interactions between these client and therapist influences can be extensive, many determining how psychotherapy progresses. We will take a look at the most relevant interactions—transference and countertransference, personality interactions, and client challenges to therapist skills—but do keep in mind the potential for diverse options, and how they might impact on the success of psychotherapy.

TRANSFERENCE AND COUNTERTRANSFERENCE

Feeling, thoughts, and behavior pertaining to individuals in the present can be derived from past relationships, referred to as transference when the client experiences it, and countertransference when the therapist reacts in this fashion to the client. Both transference and countertransference have a powerful influence on how psychotherapy progresses, amplified by interactive effects. Interactions between transference and countertransference transpire when there is the simultaneous occurrence of the client reacting to the therapist based on earlier relationships, and the therapist responding to the client on the basis of past scenarios. This adds complexity to transference and countertransference reactions, but is very understandable considering that either or both processes can and do unfold in the context of psychotherapy. I will now provide some client examples demonstrating how transference and countertransference can interact.

Considering that transference and countertransference can be negative or positive, with a range for each, there are several basic combinations: positive transference—negative countertransference, positive transference—positive

DOI: 10.4324/b23346-17

countertransference, negative transference—negative countertransference, negative transference—positive countertransference. An example of positive transference—negative countertransference is provided by John, a middle-aged waiter with significant alcohol abuse problems identifying as being homosexual. John had a history of dependent relationships derived from his insecurities and anxiety, and he demonstrated excessive reliance on his aging mother who he depended on for monetary assistance and also companionship when not in a romance. His pattern in romances consisted of a passionate start, usually fueled by alcohol, then disintegration when his partner realized how dependent he was becoming. Breakups often triggered alcohol binges that led to a few brief hospitalizations. A positive, and as it turned out erotic, transference formed early on in sessions with him seeing me as a supportive person. My countertransference was negative as I am independent by nature, and he reminded me of clingy clients and others that evoked negative feelings. I addressed his dependence and how it set up a pattern of attempted romances, failures, and intensified drinking. His response consisted on showing up intoxicated and trying to come on to me. He expressed that he found me attractive and someone that he feels close to. I struggled with my reaction in the moment because of the negative countertransference, but aware of it I was able to react objectively enough to politely assert boundaries, including no physical contact and also not showing up intoxicated. During the next session when he was sober, we used the experience to explore his dysfunctional relationship pattern that reinforced problem drinking. This intervention triggered a long stretch of him remaining sober and trying to limit his dependence in romantic relationships. As is common with addictions, he did have a couple of relapses with alcohol, but they were triggered by work setbacks and not romance issues. John's example demonstrates how it is important for therapists to be aware of their countertransference feelings, as events can occur in the moment that are pivotal to the success of psychotherapy, and unlikely to be dealt with effectively if the therapist is unaware of relevant countertransference feelings.

Positive transference—positive countertransference transpired with an early 30s client, Tony, who was depressed and anxious due to a sense that his life was not going anywhere. He worked as a technician in a sports store earning minimum wage and lived with his parents as he could not afford to live alone. Lacking confidence in himself, largely due to the career, finance, and housing limitations, he avoided romances but did have some male friends. I prescribed an antidepressant when it became clear that his anxiety and depression, combined with a pattern of avoidance, blocked him from progressing. The combination of the antidepressant and psychotherapy focused on reasonable career change, shifted him into an optimistic frame of mind. Shortly he proposed that work as an electrician excited him and we looked at how he could move toward this goal in comfortable steps. His parents were very supportive and offered to pay for the schooling involved, which further motivated him. Having struggled with high school he expressed fear of math and physics, required subjects for electrician training, but in keeping with the stepwise progression, I had him seek out online resources and start working on these challenging topics. From this effort, he realized that he could learn both, which bolstered his confidence and motivation to enroll in the necessary courses. His transference was positive based on both parents being supportive of him, even if he remained a sports technician ongoing. He expressed that he was pleased by my support of a technical career and how I mentioned that he already had good skills in this regard, as he was wary of people pushing him to a university scenario. My countertransference was positive based on having done technical work installing floors during summers when in high school and early university, and fond memories of the relationships with coworkers, particularly the humor so lacking in many settings. The mutual positive feelings provided a very supportive and stable platform for him to progress with his new career direction.

On a more negative note is a unique client example involving negative transference—negative countertransference. Earlier in my career as a psychiatrist Crystal attended for what she described as coping problems. In her early thirties, Crystal was going through a second divorce with both marriages described as quite volatile. These romance issues were probably derived from being molested by her financially successful stepfather once when he was intoxicated, and an absent biological father. In the initial sessions, I sensed a positive reaction to me but also an undercurrent of something else that was hard to pinpoint. Discussing her marriages, a pattern emerged consisting of developing a relationship with successful men, that despite being very vibrant initially, declined with substantial volatility. Her first husband was well off financially owning his own business, and her second husband turned out to be her divorce lawyer from the first marriage, who was older and very successful. Relevant to the relationship pattern, Crystal was extremely attractive and well beyond the norm of even attractive women with no physical imperfections, as her fairly revealing clothing style confirmed. Shortly I sensed that she was starting to seduce me which triggered mixed feelings, one being pleasure that such an attractive woman is interested, but more strongly repulsion. I realized that this is where transference and countertransference were interacting.

Regarding transference, Crystal was essentially destroying successful men related to anger toward her stepfather and perhaps biological father. Crystal's first husband had been taken to the proverbial cleaners by her divorce lawyer, who she ended up seducing and marrying. One can only imagine how the second divorce would look in court, with an older lawyer sleeping with and marrying his client. The judge would likely annihilate him financially. It appeared that I was up next in this negative transference, although my finances at the time could not compare to the first two. Countertransference played a key role derived from a past brief romance with an attractive woman, who initially seemed interested evident from our initial meeting: I was getting lunch in a cafeteria type restaurant and lining up I noticed this woman looking at me, and when I looked at her she smiled. I took advantage of the opportunity and approached which led to the brief relationship. At first things seemed great but going out one time I noticed her looking at other men, all attractive and dressed well as I was during our initial encounter. This woman's background was informative as she grew up in a well-off affluent family and expected to find a very successful partner. Her first marriage was to such a man and when it failed she ended up with quite a settlement, which she had essentially burned through. Negative feelings arose in me due to both the realization that I was pretty much filling a repeat role, and her entitled nature which conflicted with my more down to earth nature, as evident from installing floors during my high school and early university years. I had a real sense of let down as the early promise degenerated into "crap" for lack of a better term. Feelings about this short-lived partner surfaced with Crystal which raised the question, what to do about this negative transference—negative countertransference scenario? My response was to end the sessions with a suggestion that she see a female therapist given that she had not indicated any homosexual desires, as a female therapist would not be a target for seduction and could work more effectively with the situation. Perhaps I could have continued sessions with Crystal but the relationship was becoming heated in more ways than one, and it is often best for both parties to eject at this juncture. In addition, she would likely have been willing to discuss feelings about men more openly with a female therapist, instead of repeating the transference related pattern.

Negative transference—positive countertransference is an interesting combination, and the example of Roberto comes to mind. This young man presented with some anxiety issues and a focus on self-improvement. He had engaged in various obscure types of psychotherapy, most I had never even heard of, and really seemed motivated. He evoked a positive countertransference as he reminded me of very psychologically minded prior clients and also people like this in my life outside of psychotherapy, who really focus on self-improvement. Despite an initially promising start psychotherapy faltered and he indicated that he was ending it. Quite surprised, I questioned him and his response revealed negativity in that he viewed psychiatrists as pushing certain agendas, whereas the therapists of the more obscure forms of therapy he tried were not like this. Aware of his history with critical and successful parents, I attempted a transference interpretation, which he used to confirm his perspective that psychiatrists have their agendas. I offered that if he wished to try it again I will see him but he never rebooked. Roberto apparently had negative transference feelings about successful authority figures based on the criticisms from his parents, whereas the marginalized therapists were identified with. However, given that his issues persisted one has to wonder how effective these alternative therapies were.

The examples provided cover positive transference—negative countertransference, positive transference—positive countertransference, negative transference—negative countertransference, negative transference—positive countertransference, demonstrating how intriguing the interactions between transference and countertransference can be. Most discussions and research examining these client and therapist influences treat them in isolation from one another, an occurrence that might seem repeated here with coverage of transference and countertransference in separate chapters, but since transference is client based and countertransference therapist based, separate chapters are warranted. The inclusion of transference and countertransference interactions in this chapter highlights how truly interactive they often are.

PERSONALITY INTERACTIONS

Considering that it is quite rare for a licensed psychotherapist to have a full-fledged personality disorder, most personality interactions involve normal expressions, with the so-called Big 5 of extraversion-introversion, neurotic-emotionally stable, open-closed to experience, agreeable-antagonism, and conscientious-negligence (see the Personality Disorders chapter) most relevant. As has been mentioned neurotic-emotionally stable is really reactivity. For the most part, interactions between people are best when they share personality traits, and this applies to client and therapist interactions. For example, you might find it challenging to bond with someone who is closed to experience if you are open to experience. You suggest attending a unique music performance and the person declines, but is willing to see the currently favored pop start who bores you. Likewise, if you are very extroverted and wish to attend a social gathering, a friendship with an introverted person who only wants to see a movie with one person does not really work well. This fit, or lack thereof, plays a role in therapy interactions, as with a client who is open to experience wanting to explore their dreams, and a closed to experience therapist adhering to a manualized version of some form of therapy, or the client and therapist openness to experience reversed. The same degree of difficulty might not apply to extroversion-introversion, but will to some extent if an extroverted therapist is suggesting outgoing behavior that does not fit with a client's introverted nature, or an introverted therapist proposing more solitary activity when the extroverted client desires highly sociable activity. Similar interaction problems can arise with the conscientious-negligence dimension of normal personality, such as when a highly conscientious therapist encounters a client who does not follow through on homework assignments, and a very conscientious client wanting precise strategies that do not align with a less conscientious therapists free-flowing approach.

Regarding what can be done about these normal personality mismatches, the starting point is to understand normal personality dimensions, where you as a therapist rate, and assess clients for their approximate levels on the dimensions. Although it is more ideal to actually have this tested formally, I find it quite easy to gauge where a client rates, based on how they respond to issues in therapy and descriptions of interactions and approaches to life outside of therapy. For instance, if a person likes novel pursuits and more adventurous travel, then it is a safe bet that the person is quite high on openness to experience, but if they describe safe limited activities and travel then the individual is likely low on this dimension, unless anxiety and/or depression interferes with the expression of their natural tendency. Likewise, the degree of extroversion-introversion and conscientious-negligence is usually evident from information presented about their life and response to therapy suggestions. A client who rejects any outgoing behavior that is proposed and engages in more solitary activities is almost certainly to the introverted side of the extroversion-introversion dimension. Diligence to therapeutic tasks such as self-esteem journaling reflects conscientiousness, as do descriptions of completing work tasks.

When client and therapist align in terms of openness to experience, extroversion-introversion, and conscientiousness, the therapeutic alliance will likely proceed easier. If there are mismatches, awareness and understanding on the part of the therapist can help to compensate. For instance, setting expectations for what the client is likely to accept based on their standing with the given personality dimensions. There is no sense suggesting novel pursuits to a person who is closed to experience, although a person who is open to experience but blocked due to anxiety and/or depression might find that engaging in novel activities is a way to overcome their mental health issues. A client who is introverted will typically resist suggestions for group involvements, but if the activity is positive and productive like Toastmasters he or she might engage and benefit. Explaining the advantages and exploring fears can assist in the client's progression to the activity. Expecting a person who is low in conscientiousness to reliably complete therapy homework is setting up friction. In this instance, a less formal approach to therapy is usually the best approach.

The other two Big 5 normal personality dimensions of agreeable-antagonism and neurotic-emotionally stable (reactivity) are somewhat different, in that on the more negative side client-therapist alignment is problematic, as it is for any relationship: while agreeable-agreeable and low reactivity-low reactivity favor a good relationship, disagreeable-disagreeable and reactive-reactive often lead to friction. For instance, a disagreeable client rejecting interpretations by the therapist, and the disagreeable therapist responding negatively to the client's alternative suggestions. Therapy can rapidly deteriorate and the already disagreeable client will usually dropout. An agreeable therapist will be more willing to work with the client's resistance and roll with it, allowing the client to develop trust and respect, leading to improvements in terms of agreeableness. Likewise, an agreeable client might roll with a more opinionated therapist. When both the client and therapist are highly reactive, it is like one of those pinball machines with each bouncing off the others' input that is not clearly positive. If the therapist is less reactive then more thoughtful and measured responses to the client's over-reactions can transpire, providing the client with a template for less intense reactivity. If the therapist is highly reactive a low reactivity client might tolerate and potentially even learn from the response. As with the other normal personality dimensions, where a client rates on agreeableness and reactivity can be assessed from both interactions in therapy and examples they provide of social encounters outside of therapy. When the therapist is disagreeable and/or reactive they really do need to be aware of their normal personality profile and compensate, such as by practicing an under-standing of diverse perspectives and conciliatory statements if disagreeable, and suppressing initial responses, rethinking the situation briefly, and responding on this basis if highly reactive (SUPPRESS-THINK-RESPOND). We cannot radically alter our standing on normal personality dimensions, but through con-scious effort and practice can override and somewhat shift the profile.

Interactions between client and therapist normal personality dimensions are then very important but rarely discussed. As with relationships outside of therapy, alignment on the dimensions of open-closed to experience, extraver-sion-introversion, and conscientious-negligence works very well. Mismatches do require awareness and effort on the part of the therapist to compensate. Alignment on the negative side of the agreeable-antagonism and reactivity (neurotic-emotionally stable) dimensions are very problematic, and the thera-pist must be aware of this occurrence and actively address the issue. Fortunately, by understanding and working with normal personality dimensions, client and therapist interactions can be optimized.

CLIENT CHALLENGES TO THERAPIST SKILLS

Various client influences pertaining to psychotherapy progress interact with therapist skills, and it is important for therapists to be aware of these potential interactions and manage them. Although there are numerous feasible interac-tions of this nature, the ones that stand out consist of expectations, motivation, resistance and noncompliance, and complexity.

Expectations

The Expectation-Reality Match (or Mismatch) was discussed in the Expectations chapter. When reality falls short of expectations disappointment as a variant of sadness is typically experienced. Clients entering therapy with too high expectations are likely to be disappointed with how therapy is progressing. Perfectionistic clients are particularly prone to this but there are many sources of unrealistically high expectations. Where I quite often note this is with clients expecting depression, anxiety, and other mental health problems to be fully resolved. Another misguided expectation is that progress will be linear when it frequently follows a different course in psychotherapy: an initial gradual pro-gression followed by more rapid gains as the client advances with the man-agement of their problem. Then there are the clients who hold very negative perspectives, and based on this, doubt what psychotherapy can do for them.

These various expectation impediments to psychotherapy progress must be managed by the therapist, necessitating solid skills including understanding, communication, and rapport building. In the instance of too high expectations, the therapist needs to assist the client in resetting their expectations such that they perceive gains. This intervention must be done in a fashion that builds rapport and not be perceived as challenging. Pertaining to the excessively high expectation that the problem will fully resolve, I find it useful to comment something to the effect of, "It would be nice if problems can be fully resolved, but in medicine many issues tend to be ongoing or recurrent like asthma and headaches. Often the best we can hope for is that the problem is settled and by working together we can keep it under control." I find that clients process this well as they can place their mental health issues in the larger general health context, and the use of "we" and "together" communicates that I intend to work with the person helping to foster rapport. The expectation that progress will be linear is managed by understanding that non-linear progress is often what transpires in therapy, and expressing this concept to the client. The conceptual shift fosters patience instead of frustration and disappointment. Negative perspectives pertaining to therapy benefit from the therapist assisting the person in learning how to reframe negative views, with "assisting" very collaborative and hence rapport building. Therapist skills are then very relevant to scenarios where clients' expectations hinder the progress of therapy with understanding, communication, and rapport building paramount.

An interesting version of expectation-reality mismatch transpires when the therapist expects too much from the client. Therapists hold expectations for client progress that can be applied across the board, or to particular individuals based on features of the client or countertransference reactions. For instance, a therapist might assume that more educated clients can advance further, or a positive countertransference sets up a belief that the particular client should excel. If the client lives up to the therapist's expectations, or better yet exceeds them, then the therapist perceives a gain and feels happiness or a variant such as satisfaction. But what if the client does not live up to the expectations? Negative emotions arise often including frustration with the client and the progress of therapy, these feelings likely impairing the therapeutic alliance, in turn limiting client progression, producing more frustration on the part of the therapist, and so on. To manage excessively high expectations relative to what the client lives up to, a therapist must be aware of his or her expectations for clients, both in general and for specific individuals. If these expectations are too high, perhaps even perfectionistic, then moderation is definitely required. Recalling the crucial expectation-reality match or mismatch, and how when reality exceeds expectations a gain is perceived, will help motivate this shift. Discussions with colleagues regarding reasonable expectations for client progress can also be helpful in resetting expectations. I strongly recommend not bypassing this suggestion, because having reasonable expectations for client progress contributes to the mental wellbeing of therapists, and hence resilience to burnout.

Therapists can also have too low expectations for clients, a scenario that is often encountered with clients who have a variety of challenging presentations.

In instances of "intimidating" clients, the person is often seen as being different than the therapist setting up a divide that results in the therapist not anticipating beneficial change (Fisch & Schlanger, 1999). By not being overwhelmed by the presentation and refraining from psychologically distancing oneself from the client, the therapist can assist the client in making positive change even in a brief psychotherapy context (Fisch & Schlanger, 1999). Believing in the possibility of change with such clients is important in engaging effectively and overcoming any resistance derived from the "intimidating" presentation (Fisch & Schlanger, 1999). When therapists manage their own expectations for client improvement and communicate appropriate expectations to the client progress is enhanced, even in very short-term therapy consisting of a few sessions (Battino, 2006).

Motivation

Given that therapists are typically highly motivated to provide psychotherapy, motivation problems are usually client based. There is an interaction issue given that the therapist is motivated whereas the client is insufficiently motivated. Client motivation problems include: benefits of therapy are perceived as less than costs, limited intrinsic motivation, and insufficient change motivation (see the Motivation chapter). Since therapists are not salespeople it takes skill to promote the benefits of therapy without selling it. Reviewing with the client the realistic benefits covered in the Motivation chapter and exploring the costs that they perceive, can help reset the balance in favor of benefits. Limitations with intrinsic motivation often occur in the context of the client being forced or pressured to attend. Having the client consider the broader scope of possible benefits beyond the source motivating attendance, instills a sense of choice that increases motivation. Communication skill is required because the client might perceive you the therapist as one more extrinsic source of motivation, further reducing any perception of control.

Insufficient change motivation arises from various sources including closed to experience as a personality trait, fear of change, and rigid patterns of behavior. The skill of recognizing normal personality traits was covered under Personality Interactions. By framing change in a safe stepwise fashion even very closed to experience clients can find the motivation to change. Fear of change leads to avoidance behavior blocking progress, and successfully managing avoidance is a refined psychotherapy skill. Regarding fear of psychotherapy, exploration of client's concerns about therapy can reduce fears and avoidance. Covering how facing fears typically results in reduced anxiety and when done in small steps there is little risk, can further overcome fear thereby instilling motivation. Rapport building helps the client feel that they are not alone in this challenge. Rigid dysfunctional patterns of behavior block positive change, and must be identified and assertively addressed by the therapist requiring confidence and direct communication. Given that the dysfunctional behavior is a default pattern, it will resurface necessitating vigilance and ongoing input from the therapist.

Client motivation problems often result in psychotherapy failing to progress with the client dropping out. Perceived costs > benefits and/or impaired intrinsic motivation create obstacles right from the start. Insufficient change motivation in terms of closed to experience, fear and avoidance, and dysfunctional patterns of behavior impedes ongoing progress with psychotherapy. By applying interpersonal and other skills therapists can improve a client's motivation such that they engage with therapy and persevere.

Resistance and Noncompliance

There are several sources of client resistance and noncompliance that limit the progress of psychotherapy, including emotional, dysfunctional patterns of behavior, personality disorder issues, and negative transference (see the Resistance and Noncompliance chapter). I will not review these here but generally indicate that psychotherapy skills are crucial if the block is to be eliminated or reduced. For instance, with emotional blocks such as fear, anger, guilt, and shame, the therapist must feel and understand the emotional perspective of the client (empathy) and build rapport, such that the person feels supported in resolving the emotional suffering. Ambivalence is common when emotions are involved since $+3$ and -3 coexist creating a dissonant state. Appreciating when clients are ambivalent and assisting in resolution of the dissonance, combined with developing tolerance for some ambivalence if less intense, are more advanced skills that optimize the progress of psychotherapy. In the instance of dysfunctional patterns of behavior, a therapist needs to identify the source, either an internalized pattern of behavior from caregivers or trauma related, as the interventions differ: guiding and encouraging the client to consciously practice alternative more constructive behavior for internalized dysfunctional patterns of behavior, and process trauma by grieving losses associated with it to fuse the dissociated emotional and cognitive components. Therapist skills are really put to the test when it comes to personality disorder sources of resistance and noncompliance, with self-support being very important. Recognizing and managing negative transference is crucial for preventing therapy ruptures and assisting clients in managing issues from their past. Limited and high probability transference interpretations (quality over quantity) is the best option for managing negative transference. Marriage of client resistance and noncompliance to robust therapist skills removes blocks and fosters progress.

Complexity

In the Complexity chapter, we looked at how comorbidity per se does not limit psychotherapy, but this is based on the assumption that the therapist has the skills required to assess and address comorbid conditions present in a diversity of clients. If skills such as rapport building and communication are lacking, then progress might well be impeded. Likewise, techniques for managing depression, anxiety, personality disorders, and the range of mental health problems, are crucial. Severity is a consideration independent of comorbidity that really does limit outcomes, even when therapist skills are robust. Clients with severe expressions of any mental illness are more challenging to manage. I am fortunate in that medication is part of what I offer, because severe manifestations usually do require a combination of psychotherapy and medications. However, with personality disorders medications are of limited value unless there is comorbid depression, intense anxiety, or psychosis. Therapist skills interact with client comorbidity and severity, and really put these skills, including self-support, to the test.

SUMMARY NOTE

Interactions between client and therapist influences can be almost as extensive as the imagination and experience reveals. The focus here has been on the most potent consisting of: transference and countertransference, personality factors (normal personality traits), and client challenges to therapist skills covering expectations, motivation, resistance and noncompliance, and complexity. Therapist skills acquired through experience, readings, and training, really do make a difference in the management of these challenging interactions. Ultimately, via empathy, communication, rapport building, techniques, and even organizational skills to run an effective psychotherapy practice, challenging interactions between client and therapist influences can be shifted from potential or actual blocks to solid progress and good outcomes.

REFERENCES

Battino, R. (2006). *Expectation: The very brief therapy book*. Crown House Publishing.

Fisch, R., & Schlanger, K. (1999). *Brief therapy with intimidating cases: Changing the unchangeable*. Jossey-Bass.

CONCLUDING WORD

To optimize psychotherapy progress impediments must be identified and effectively addressed. These blocks involve client, therapist, and interactive influences as psychotherapy is ultimately a relationship. Client influences that can impede progress include: motivation, expectations, personality disorders, reinforcement parameters, complexity, resistance and noncompliance, impaired states and processes for mental health, and transference. Therapist influences consist of: countertransference, emotional factors, personality factors, and skill factors. Interactive involve the therapeutic alliance and various interactions between client and therapist influences, such as transference and countertransference, normal personality, and client challenges to therapist skills (expectations, motivation, resistance and noncompliance, and complexity). As with any involved process it is challenging to disentangle the various influences, but the divisions applied do align with clinical experience and research. In addition to the comprehensive client, therapist, and interactive influences coverage, there are several strengths to the approach taken that translate into effective management of blocks and hindrances to the progress of psychotherapy.

Most treatments of the topic work from a set theoretical perspective. While some issues might apply more to one type of therapy, as with homework to cognitive therapy, impediments to the progress of psychotherapy span all types of therapy, every form of mental illness, and diverse clients. For example, transference that historically has been linked to psychoanalysis, spans the mental illness and client spectrum ensuring that it is involved in all types of therapy. The approach taken is not rooted in any one theoretical perspective, and the strategies to manage the impediments reflect this orientation, being applicable to all types of therapy, all mental illness manifestations, and with diverse clients.

Relevant to the issue of types of therapy and how psychotherapy actually works, instead of the special sauce of a given form of therapy, it appears that psychotherapy advances key states and processes for mental health (activity, psychological defense mechanisms, social connectedness, psychological regulation, human specific cognition, self-acceptance, and adaptability). This across therapy perspective encompasses non-specific factors such as behavioral activation and hope as they also advance the states and processes for mental health, providing an explanation for why they are so effective in a psychotherapy universe dominated by specific forms of therapy. Coverage of the states and processes for mental health, and how impairments to them impede both mental health and psychotherapy, is unique, and provides an additional way for psychotherapists to view and address both mental illness and barriers to psychotherapy progress.

Many articles and books pertaining to psychotherapy impediments emphasize resistance and noncompliance, or on a slightly more positive note, ambivalence. I believe that most clients have the potential to substantially improve with psychotherapy, and if this is not materializing then something must be interfering or blocking it. This much more positive perspective than resistance, noncompliance, and ambivalence, is in my opinion accurate based on extensive psychotherapy experience, and generates optimism that progress can transpire if the impediments are understood and addressed. The coverage of client, therapist, and interactive influences, provides therapists with the knowledge and practical skills required to manage the many issues that can impede psychotherapy progress.

Given that the client plays a major role in why psychotherapy does not progress, it makes sense to provide strategies for the client that will assist in reducing or removing the impediment. Most treatments of the topic, though, only emphasize what the therapist can do about the client's problem. The inclusion here of what clients can do, where relevant, assists in addressing impediments to psychotherapy progress as this approach gives the client an active and empowering role.

Consistent with the power of relationships derived from our social evolution, psychotherapy is the most common and significant intervention when the full spectrum of mental illness is considered. Even for psychosis that is typically viewed as only the domain of medication treatments, psychotherapy is effective. Hence, it is important to appreciate the value of psychotherapy and do everything reasonably possible to remove impediments. With the knowledge and strategies relevant to client, therapist, and interactive influences provided here, progress can be optimized allowing psychotherapy to achieve its full potential.

INDEX